Pleural Diseases

Clinical Cases and Real-World Discussions

CLAUDIO SORINO, MD, PhD
Division of Pulmonary and Critical Care Medicine
Sant'Anna Hospital
Como, Italy

DAVID FELLER-KOPMAN, MD, FCCP
Division of Pulmonary and Critical Care Medicine
Johns Hopkins University
Baltimore, Maryland, United States

GIAMPIETRO MARCHETTI, MD, FCCP
Division of Pulmonary and Critical Care Medicine
Spedali Civili
Brescia, Italy

ELSEVIER Philadelphia, PA

ELSEVIER

1600 John F. Kennedy Blvd.
Ste 1800
Philadelphia, PA 19103-2899

PLEURAL DISEASES: CLINICAL CASES AND REAL-WORLD   ISBN: 978-0-323795418
DISCUSSIONS

Front cover image by Domenico Loizzi

Library of Congress Control Number: 2020949330

Content Strategist: Robin Carter
Content Development Specialist: Meghan Andress
Publishing Services Manager: Shereen Jameel
Senior Project Manager: Kamatchi Madhavan
Design Direction: Renee Duenow

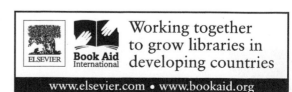

Working together
to grow libraries in
developing countries

www.elsevier.com • www.bookaid.org

Printed in the United States of America

Last digit is the print number: 9   8   7   6   5   4   3   2   1

ACKNOWLEDGMENTS

The editors thank Dr. Agazio Francesco Ussia and Dr. Andrea Tironi for their contributions to anatomic pathological issues; Dr. Maurizio Manara for providing interesting radiological images; Dr. Alessandra Butti for her suggestions on nephrological issues; Dr. Natalia Buda for reviewing ultrasound images and their description and Dr. Maria Teresa Congedo for the video on the chest drain insertion using the Seldinger technique.

PREFACE

It was June 2015 when a group of doctors from the Spedali Civili of Brescia, Italy, created the first social network dedicated to the study of pleural diseases, called Pleural-HUB. In a short time, it has become a virtual place to share curiosities about the pleura, discuss the mechanisms of the pathologies that affect it, and compare the possible methods for diagnosis and treatment.

Today the group has over 5000 members from all over the world. They include professors, researchers, clinicians, young doctors in training, nurses, and physiotherapists, all willing to get involved and share their experiences and uncertainties.

The progressive growth of the group and its activities represent the expression of a widespread desire for knowledge in a field of medicine that has been underappreciated for a long time. Pleural diseases often occupy a small part of books on respiratory disorders, even though pleural diseases are commonly found in medical practice, especially by pulmonologists, internists, oncologists, radiologists, and thoracic surgeons.

The Pleural-HUB group has become a tool through which many clinicians ask for help in dealing with complicated cases, quickly obtaining an exchange of views among dozens of doctors from different teams and different hospital contexts.

In addition to its immediate clinical use, this approach is extremely didactic and has led us to the idea of collecting some cases and presenting them together with the discussions that doctors carried out in the real world.

The project, initially called "Pleural disease in real-life" was quite ambitious. Thanks to the extensive network of collaborations, the work was pleasant and rewarding on many occasions.

The COVID-19 pandemic hindered the writing of the book as many of us for several months were involved in the front-line fight against the SARS-CoV-2 that is devastating all of humanity. Despite this, we managed to move forward with this book and we are proud of the result.

This book includes three groupings of pleural diseases: malignancies, infectious diseases, and miscellaneous. A large portion of space was reserved for discussion on thoracic ultrasound, an indispensable method for studying the pleura today. Minimally invasive procedures are widely addressed, such as thoracentesis, placement of thoracic tubes, and thoracoscopy.

This book is organized as a collection of clinical cases of patients with pleural disease or injury, who were managed in respiratory care units. The description of each case includes the onset of symptoms, the entire diagnostic-therapeutic path, and discussions on the clinical choices made. The chapters do not describe the best approach possible but what doctors did in certain circumstances. Our aim was to introduce the readers to medical real-life cases, allowing them to remember important clinical lessons and even to learn from errors. A focus on the most relevant issues is also present.

In addition to the management of pleural diseases, common clinical issues are addressed, such as the management of older patients with multiple morbidities, the optimization of fluid balance, and the need to discontinue antiplatelet or anticoagulant therapy before invasive procedures.

A rich iconography embellishes the pages of this volume. We hope that it will be appreciated and considered educational by readers. Our hope is that readers will feel like virtual attending physicians and will be stimulated by the clinical reasoning.

We thank many doctors, including Dr. Tiziana Cappelletti, Dr. Giuseppe Milani, and Dr. Antonio Raco, who provided their support during the long process that gave birth to the current version of the book.

The book is dedicated to all patients who have died from pleural diseases and to all healthcare professionals who have devotedly worked during the COVID-19 outbreak.

Claudio Sorino

David Feller-Kopman

Giampietro Marchetti

CONTRIBUTORS

Sergio Agati, MD
Division of Pulmonary and Critical Care
 Medicine
Sant'Anna Hospital
Como, Italy

Pietro Bertoglio, MD
Division of Thoracic Surgery
IRCCS Sacro Cuore Don Calabria Hospital
Cancer Care Centre Negrar
Verona, Italy

Natalia Buda, MD, PhD
Department of Internal Medicine, Connective
 Tissue Diseases and Geriatrics
Medical University of Gdansk
Gdansk, Poland

Angelo Calati, MD
Division of Thoracic Surgery
Sant'Anna Hospital
Como, Italy

Paolo Carlucci, MD
Respiratory Unit, Department of Health
 Sciences
San Paolo Hospital, University of Milan
Milan, Italy

Stefano Elia
Division of Radiology
Hospital of Esine (BG)
Esine, Italy

David Feller-Kopman, MD, FCCP
Johns Hopkins University
Division of Pulmonary and Critical Care
 Medicine
Baltimore, Maryland, United States

Hari Kishan Gonuguntla, MD, DM
Division of Interventional Pulmonology
Yashoda Hospitals
Hyderabad, India

Nitesh Gupta, MD, DM
Division of Pulmonary and Critical Care
 Medicine
VMMC – Safdarjung Hospital
New Delhi, India

Alraiyes Abdul Hamid, MD, FCCP
Department of Pulmonary, Critical Care and
 Sleep Medicine
Rosalind Franklin University of Medicine and
 Science
North Chicago, Illinois, United States

Francesco Inzirillo, MD
Department of Thoracic Surgery
Morelli Hospital, AOVV
Sondalo (SO), Italy

Filippo Lococo, MD, PhD
Thoracic Unit
Catholic University of the Sacred Heart
Rome, Italy

Giampietro Marchetti, MD, FCCP
Division of Pulmonary and Critical Care
 Medicine
Spedali Civili
Brescia, Italy

Fabrizio Minervini, MD, PhD
Department of Thoracic Surgery
Cantonal Hospital Lucerne
Lucerne, Switzerland

Michele Mondoni, MD
Respiratory Unit, Department of Health
 Sciences
San Paolo Hospital, University of Milan
Milan, Italy

Stefano Negri, MD
Division of Pulmonary and Critical Care
 Medicine
Sant'Anna Hospital
Como, Italy

Giuseppe Pepe, MD
Division of Pulmonary and Critical Care
  Medicine
Guido Salvini Hospital, Garbagnate Milanese
Milan, Italy

Valentina Pinelli, MD
Division of Pulmonology
San Bartolomeo Hospital
Sarzana (La Spezia), Italy

Fabio Pirracchio, MD
University of Milan
Department of Pathophysiology and
  Transplantation
Milan, Italy

Fondazione IRCCS Ca' Granda Ospedale
Maggiore Policlinico
Respiratory Unit and Cystic Fibrosis Adult
  Center
Milan, Italy

Cecilia Sampietro, MD
Division of Thoracic Surgery
Sant'Anna Hospital
Como, Italy

Marco Scarci, MD
Department of Thoracic Surgery
San Gerardo Hospital
Monza, Italy

Claudio Sorino, MD, PhD
Division of Pulmonary and Critical Care
  Medicine
Sant'Anna Hospital
Como, Italy

Mario Spatafora, MD, PhD
Biomedical Department of Internal and
  Specialist Medicine
University of Palermo
Palermo, Italy

Alessandro Squizzato, MD, PhD
Research Centre on Thromboembolic
  Diseases and Antithrombotic Therapies
Department of Medicine and Surgery,
  University of Insubria
Varese and Como, Italy

Mario Tamburrini, MD
Pulmonology Unit
Azienda Sanitaria Friuli Occidentale
Pordenone, Italy

Alessandro Zanforlin, MD, PhD
Pulmonology Service
Azienda Sanitaria dell'Alto Adige
Bolzano, Italy

CONTENTS

VIDEO CONTENTS

PART I

Malignancies

Malignant Pleural Effusion With Nonexpandable Lung and Hydropneumothorax After ▶ Thoracentesis

Claudio Sorino ■ David Feller-Kopman ■ Giampietro Marchetti

History of Present Illness

A 60-year-old Caucasian man presented to the hospital with shortness of breath and right lateral chest pain. These symptoms had begun about a month earlier, after a flu-like episode with cough and low-grade fever, and had progressively worsened. Chest radiography, requested by the primary care physician, had revealed right-sided pleural effusion, without shift of the mediastinum (Fig. 1.1). Consequently an urgent referral to the pulmonology department was made.

Past Medical History

The patient was a truck driver, current smoker of about 40 cigarettes a day, with a 70-pack-year history of smoking. He had not had any asbestos exposure, no known risk factors for tuberculosis, and no history of drug abuse, weight loss, or anorexia. He had never undergone pulmonary function tests. He took daily medications for hypercholesterolemia (simvastatin).

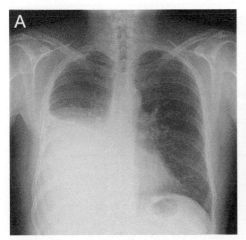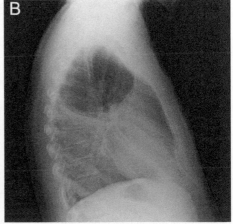

Fig. 1.1 Posteroanterior (A) and lateral (B) chest radiographs showing large right pleural effusion, without mediastinal shift.

Physical Examination and Early Clinical Findings

At the time of the visit to the pulmonologist, the patient was afebrile (body temperature 36.7° C [98.06 °F]), alert, and cooperative. Oxygen saturation measured by pulse oximetry was 97% on room air, heart rate was 80 beats/min, respiratory rate was 23 breaths/min, and blood pressure was 130/85 mm Hg.

On chest examination, the breath sounds were absent in the infrascapular and infra-axillary areas on the right side, and decreased fremitus and dullness to percussion were observed. No pallor, clubbing, and peripheral edema were apparent. Chest ultrasonography showed large, hypoechoic, right-sided pleural effusion, with a flattened diaphragm and paradoxical diaphragmatic motion.

Discussion Topic

Pulmonologist A

Extraction and analysis of pleural fluid are necessary to identify the cause of pleural effusion.

Pulmonologist B

Thoracoscopy would allow for exploration of the pleural cavity and performance of pleural biopsies. However, we could achieve the diagnosis in a less invasive way. Placement of a thoracic drainage tube is probably a good choice in view of the abundant amount of fluid in the pleural cavity.

Pulmonologist A

Why not consider thoracentesis as the first step? We can perform it in a short time as an outpatient procedure.

Pulmonologist B

We also need a chest computed tomography because it can help properly evaluate the lung parenchyma.

Pulmonologist A

I suggest performing the chest CT after pleural fluid removal. This would allow for a better view of both the lung parenchyma and the pleura. Moreover, thanks to ultrasound guidance, thoracentesis is very safe even without CT.

Recent blood tests had shown a hemoglobin level of 15.4 g/dL and total leukocyte count of 9,720 cells/mm³, with a normal differential count. The platelet count was 150,000 cells/μL, the international normalized ratio (INR) was 1.06. After injection of a local anesthetic (2% lidocaine), right thoracentesis was performed by inserting a 15-gauge Verres needle catheter connected to a

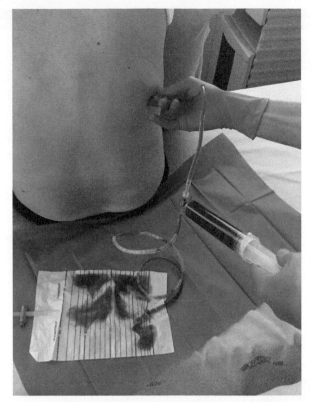

Fig. 1.2   Right thoracentesis with bloody pleural fluid.

tube with a three-way stopcock and a 2-L collecting bag. Hemorrhagic pleural fluid came out and was retained for analysis (Fig. 1.2). The procedure was well tolerated: the patient had no cough, and oxygen saturation increased to 99% during the thoracentesis. Thus a large amount of fluid (1500 mL) was extracted with the aim of achieving alleviation of symptoms and getting a better view of the lung parenchyma at the subsequent chest computed tomography (CT) scan. To facilitate removal of the liquid, slight suction was applied by means of a syringe. Toward the end of the procedure, however, the patient reported some mild, anterior chest discomfort, and after removal of another 120 mL of fluid, free aspiration of air was obtained in the syringe. Ultrasonography after the procedure revealed right-sided hydropneumothorax (Fig. 1.3), which was confirmed with chest radiography (Fig. 1.4).

Discussion Topic

How is it possible that air entered the pleural cavity? The thoracentesis was performed well. I'm sure the needle did not pierce the lung.

Pulmonologist A

Continued

Pulmonologist B

It may be that the lung does not expand properly.

Thoracic surgeon

A manometry would have helped understand if the removal of the liquid was generating a very negative intrapleural pressure. This happens if the lung is nonexpandable.

Pulmonologist A

If so, placing a chest drainage tube may not be necessary.

Thoracic surgeon

I believe that a chest tube is useful to evaluate the possibility of lung expansion.

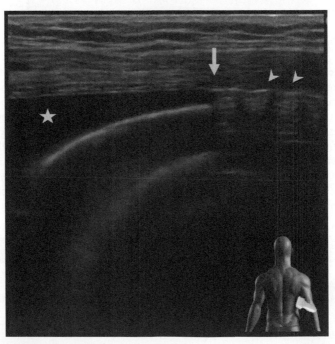

Fig. 1.3 Chest ultrasonography image showing a *double level sign* with a gas–liquid interface caused by hydropneumothorax. *Arrow,* boundary between pneumothorax and pleural effusion; *star,* anechoic pleural effusion; *arrowheads,* pneumothorax chamber.

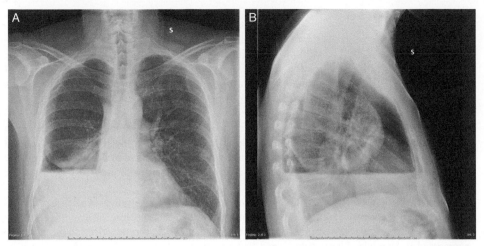

Fig. 1.4 Posteroanterior (A) and lateral (B) chest radiographs after thoracentesis showing right hydropneumo-thorax with evident air–liquid level and partial lung collapse.

A 14-French (Fr) chest drainage tube was inserted through the right fourth intercostal space. Subsequent chest CT before and after administration of iodinated contrast medium (Fig. 1.5) confirmed the presence of right hydropneumothorax that had not resolved despite placement of the chest tube. A parenchymal hypodense area suggestive for pathological solid tissue was detected in the right lower perihilar area, in correspondence with the apical segment of the inferior lobe. Some mediastinal lymph nodes were detected in the right hilar area, with a maximum diameter of about 8 mm. Finally, the postcontrast phase revealed multiple thromboembolic defects at the branches of the left pulmonary artery. This finding led to the initiation of anticoagulant injection therapy (enoxaparin subcutaneously 6000 units two times daily). The patient was admitted to the pulmonology department.

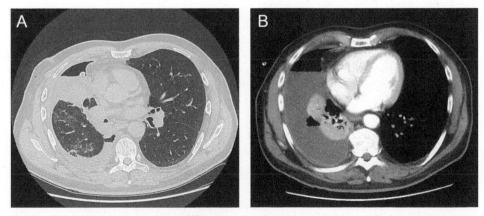

Fig. 1.5 Chest computed tomography (CT) images after chest tube positioning confirming right hydropneu-mothorax. Axial CT scan on the lung window setting (A) shows a clear air–fluid level. The chest tube is visible in the air context. Axial contrast-enhanced CT scan on the mediastinal window (B) shows pathological solid tissue in the right lower perihilar area.

Clinical Course

Pleural fluid analysis was consistent with exudative effusion: total protein was 4.5 g/dL, and lactate dehydrogenase (LDH) was 911 units/L. Patient risk factors, in particular the strong exposure to cigarette smoke, together with the appearance of the pleural fluid, were highly suspicious of malignant effusion. The hydropneumothorax was thought to be the consequence of a tumor that caused difficulty in reexpansion of the lung.

2-Deoxy-2-[fluorine-18]fluoro-D-glucose (^{18}F-FDG) PET/CT was performed (Fig. 1.6) and showed significant FDG uptake in the right hilar area, corresponding to the lesion in the apical segment of the inferior lobe (maximum standard uptake value [SUV] 8.2) and uptake in the right hilar lymph node (maximum SUV 5.2). These findings supported the hypothesis of cancer in the lower lobe of the right lung, with ipsilateral hilar lymph node metastasis.

Three slides by cytocentrifugation and nine paraffin blocks were prepared with the pleural fluid. Cytology was positive for malignancy, with evidence of atypical epithelial elements (BerEp4, an epithelial marker, was positive; calretinin, a mesothelial marker, was negative); some cells were aggregated in glandular-like structures and had cytoplasmic vacuolization, as in mucosecretion (negative Alcian-Pas). The morphological aspect and the immunophenotypic profile (napsin positive; weak focal positivity for thyroid transcription factor 1 [TTF1]) suggested adenocarcinoma of pulmonary origin.

The extent of the disease, in particular, the pleural involvement, precluded curative surgical therapy; however, systemic treatment could be undertaken. To obtain adequate neoplastic typing, with molecular profiling (epidermal growth factor receptor [EGFR] mutations, anaplastic lymphoma kinase [ALK] translocations, reactive oxygen species [ROS] rearrangements, programmed death ligand-1 [PD-L1] protein expression, see the "Focus on" box in Chapter 3), further procedures for histological sampling were considered appropriate. Bronchoscopy did not show any significant alteration of the bronchial mucosa. Blind transbronchial biopsies were performed, with no evidence of neoplastic tissue in the analyzed samples. Finally, the patient underwent video-assisted thoracoscopic surgery (VATS) of the right lung, along with multiple parietal pleural biopsies (Fig. 1.7). Tenacious pleuropulmonary adhesions were found, and mechanical lysis was attempted. However, the lower and middle lobes were nonexpandable and were not able to reoccupy the lower half of the pleural cavity; as a consequence, pleurodesis was not practicable.

At the same time, a permanent indwelling 15-Fr pleural drainage catheter with a subcutaneous access port was placed (Figs. 1.8 and 1.9) to facilitate home care and chronic management of malignant pleural effusion in a nonexpandable lung.

The postoperative course was uneventful. The histological result of the pleural biopsies was metastatic localization of lung adenocarcinoma (TTF1+, napsin A+). The percentage of tumor cells showing membrane immunoreactivity for PD-L1 (tumor proportion score [TPS]) was 60%.

Recommended Therapy and Further Indications at Discharge

The patient was discharged with a prescription for analgesic therapy (paracetamol) and anticoagulant injection (enoxaparin).

The oncologist proposed treatment with pembrolizumab, a targeted therapy recently approved as first-line monotherapy for metastatic non–small cell lung carcinoma (NSCLC) in adults whose tumors express PD-L1 with 50% or greater TPS and no EGFR- or ALK-positive tumor mutations.

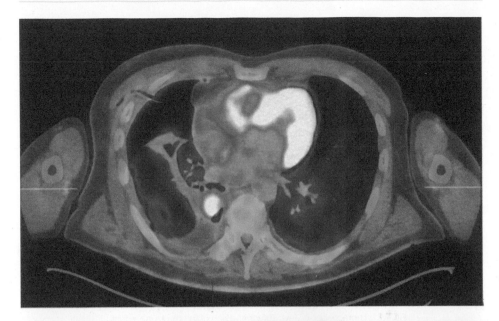

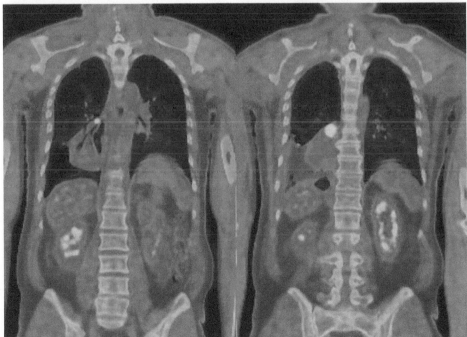

Fig. 1.6 Positron emission tomography/computed tomography (PET/CT) scan showing hyperaccumulation of the radiopharmaceutical in the apical segment of the lower lobe and in a right hilar lymph node.

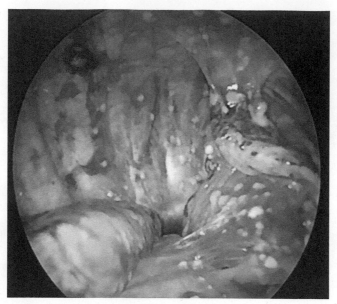

Fig. 1.7   Thoracoscopic view. Tumor invasion of the pleura is evident.

Follow-Up and Outcomes

It was recommended that the pleural catheter be drained daily through puncture of the subcutaneous port connected to the indwelling pleural catheter, and the patient experienced significant improvement in his dyspnea.

The patient received pembrolizumab at a fixed dose of 200 mg every 3 weeks. Progression-free survival was confirmed after 3 months of therapy. The oncologist proposed continuation of the

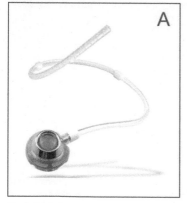 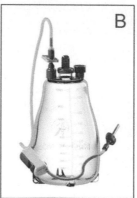 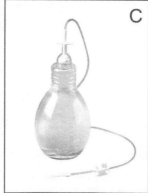

Fig. 1.8   A pleural access port system consisting of a titanium access port with a reservoir connected to a single-lumen silicone catheter reaching the pleural space. The port has a self-sealing membrane through which a particular needle (Huber noncoring needle) can be inserted to drain further liquid intermittently (A). This set-up is less commonly used compared with standard indwelling pleural catheters, such as Rocket (B) or PleurX (C).

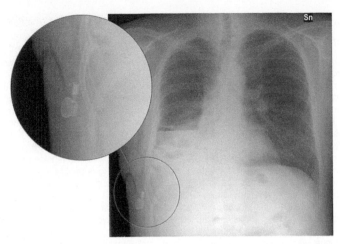

Fig. 1.9 Posteroanterior (PA) chest radiograph showing the pleural port system positioned on the right side.

drug until disease progression or unacceptable toxicity or for up to 24 months if there was no disease progression.

Focus On

Management of Malignant Pleural Effusion

Malignant pleural effusion can be caused by hematogenous or lymphatic spread of tumor cells into the pleural cavity, direct invasion of the pleura by adjacent tumors of the lung, breast, or chest wall or by cancer of the pleura itself (mesothelioma).

The indication for treatment of malignant pleural effusion is the presence of symptoms, mainly dyspnea.

The strategies to manage malignant pleural effusion depend primarily on the speed of reaccumulation of liquid and on the patient's prognosis.

One or more thoracentesis procedures may be the only choice in patients with slow reaccumulation of fluid and a poor performance status or a very limited life expectancy.

The insertion of a chest tube into the pleural cavity (thoracostomy) involves risks and morbidity, which can be justified only if survival of at least 1 month is expected.

For patients with expected survival greater than 2 to 3 months, pleurodesis or indwelling pleural catheter (IPC) placement should be considered.

Pleurodesis involves the application of a slightly irritating agent to the opposing pleural surfaces to induce their adhesion. The presence of an expandable lung, which allows the visceral and parietal pleurae to have a large contact area, is the prerequisite for the success of pleurodesis. Talc is one of the agents most commonly used for chemical pleurodesis because of its effectiveness, low cost, and easy availability.

Pleurodesis can be performed either in the form of poudrage (application of an aerosolized agent during a thoracoscopic procedure) or slurry (bedside introduction of a suspension with the irritant agent, usually with a local anesthetic, through a chest tube).

Thoracoscopy can be performed by surgeons (i.e., video-assisted thoracoscopic surgery [VATS]) or pulmonologists (i.e., medical thoracoscopy). Thoracoscopy can help in diagnosis by providing additional tissue for tumor markers or programmed death ligand-1 (PD-L1), dividing loculations when present, confirming lung re-expansion, and facilitating pleurodesis, if appropriate.

The placement of an IPC is a valid alternative to pleurodesis and is practicable as an outpatient procedure, providing similar symptom relief and improved quality of life for the patient. Unlike pleurodesis, IPC placement is an effective option to relieve dyspnea in patients with expandable or nonexpandable lung. IPC is the preferred option when the lung is unable to expand against the chest wall because pleurodesis will not be successful in this setting. The use of an IPC requires intermittent drainage by the patient or the caregiver.

Focus On

Causes of Pneumothorax After Thoracentesis

Pneumothorax is the most common complication of thoracentesis. Ultrasound guidance reduces its incidence from greater than 12% to less than 3%.

The following are the main mechanisms driving the formation of pneumothorax after thoracentesis.

- *Laceration of the visceral pleura surface by the needle or the plastic catheter.* This may be caused by excessive penetration or inadequate site of insertion, especially if the lungs are emphysematous. It occurs rarely with ultrasound-guided placement and the use of safety devices, such as Verres needles.
- *Inadvertent entry of air into the pleural cavity through the catheter.* Usually this causes pneumothorax that is of no clinical significance and that does not evolve into tension pneumothorax.
- *Pneumothorax ex vacuo.* This occurs if the underlying lung is unable to expand, for example, as a result of visceral pleural thickening, bronchial obstruction, or diseases that make the lung noncompliant (e.g., cancer or fibrosis).

In such circumstances, the pleural cavity is filled with fluid as a consequence of the negative pressure generated by an at least partially collapsed lung that is unable to expand. The removal of a large amount of pleural fluid generates negative intrapleural pressure, which can draw air from the atmosphere or from the lungs, with possible transitory opening of small visceral pleural defects.

For these reasons, pneumothorax ex vacuo often is asymptomatic, does not lead to tension pneumothorax, and does not benefit from placement of a thoracic drainage tube.

Pleural manometry during thoracentesis may reduce the risk of pneumothorax ex vacuo, allowing interruption of fluid withdrawal if the pleural pressure becomes more negative than -20 centimeters of water (cm H_2O).

Focus On

Focus on: The Nonexpandable Lung

The inability of the lung to expand to the chest wall ("nonexpandable lung") may be a mechanical complication of pleural disease, endobronchial obstruction resulting in lobar collapse, or parenchymal disease.

When the cause is a remote pleural disease, the term *trapped lung* is often used. In these circumstances, the development of a fibrous membrane around the lung impedes its expansion. Fluid removal through thoracentesis can lead to a pneumothorax ex vacuo, and the procedure may evoke chest discomfort caused by dropping pleural pressure. The use of pleural manometry may allow for diagnosis of nonexpandable lung through detection of excessive negative intrapleural pressure and of pleural elastance curves.

When nonexpandable lung is consequent to active pleural inflammation, malignancy, or hemothorax, the term *lung entrapment* is preferred. In this setting, chest radiography can show contralateral mediastinal shift, whereas pleural fluid analysis typically shows an exudate with an increase in both protein and lactate dehydrogenase (LDH). Discordant protein and LDH exudates may indicate that the inflammatory process is resolving. The presence of lung entrapment caused by malignancy reduces the possibility of successful pleurodesis.

LEARNING POINTS

- Ultrasound guidance and excellent technique minimize the development of pneumothorax after thoracentesis.
- Manometry may reduce the complication of large volume thoracentesis; however, it may be preferable not to extract greater than 1500 mL of pleural fluid.
- Small-volume thoracentesis reduces the risk of pneumothorax ex vacuo but may prevent identification of the underlying problem (i.e., underlying tumor, expandable lung) and will not offer the patient relief of their dyspnea.
- Pneumothorax ex vacuo typically does not require chest tube placement.
- Indwelling pleural catheters (IPCs) or talc pleurodesis should be considered for patients with symptomatic recurrent malignant pleural effusion. IPCs are the treatment of choice for patients with nonexpandable lung.

Further Reading

1. Huggins JT, Maldonado F, Chopra A, Rahman N, Light R. Unexpandable lung from pleural disease. *Respirology.* 2018;23(2):160–167.
2. Huggins JT, Doelken P, Sahn SA. The unexpandable lung. *Med Rep.* 2010;2:77.
3. Grabczak EM, Krenke R, Zielinska-Krawczyk M, Light RW. Pleural manometry in patients with pleural diseases—the usefulness in clinical practice. *Respir Med.* 2018;136:21–28.
4. Wahidi MM, Reddy C, Yarmus L, et al. Randomized trial of pleural fluid drainage frequency in patients with malignant pleural effusions. The ASAP trial. *Am J Respir Crit Care Med.* 2017;195(8):1050–1057.
5. Thomas R, Fysh ETH, Smith NA, et al. Effect of an indwelling pleural catheter vs talc pleurodesis on hospitalization days in patients with malignant pleural effusion: the AMPLE randomized clinical trial. *JAMA.* 2017;318(19):1903–1912.
6. Alraiyes AH, Harris K, Gildea TR. When should an indwelling pleural catheter be considered for malignant pleural effusion. *Cleve Clin J Med.* 2016;83(12):891–894.
7. Somasundaram A, Burns TF. Pembrolizumab in the treatment of metastatic non-small-cell lung cancer: patient selection and perspectives. *Lung Cancer (Auckl).* 2017;8:1–11.
8. Sul J, Blumenthal GM, Jiang X, et al. FDA approval summary: pembrolizumab for the treatment of patients with metastatic non-small cell lung cancer whose tumors express programmed death-ligand 1. *Oncologist.* 2016;21(5):643–650.

CHAPTER 2

Pleural Plaques and Malignant Pleural Mesothelioma in a Patient With Previous Asbestos Exposure

Giampietro Marchetti ■ Claudio Sorino ■ David Feller-Kopman

History of Present Illness

A 67-year-old Caucasian man went to his general practitioner because of mild exertional dyspnea. Physical examination revealed reduction in respiratory sounds in the lower right hemithorax. Chest radiography showed homogeneous right opacity with blunting of the costophrenic angle, suggestive of pleural effusion (Fig. 2.1). Empiric antibiotic therapy (amoxicillin 1 g two times daily) was prescribed for a week. One month later, chest radiography showed unchanged findings. The patient was then sent to the pulmonology department and admitted for further investigations.

Past Medical History

The patient did not have any prior medical problems and was a lifetime nonsmoker. About 30 years earlier, he had worked for about 3 years as a carpenter in close contact with flaked asbestos leaves; later he had worked as a plumber for 30 years, with possible further sporadic contact with asbestos. No family members had respiratory diseases. The patient did not routinely take any drugs.

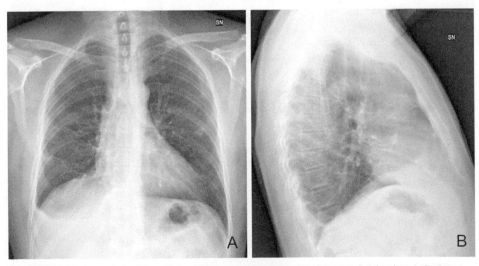

Fig. 2.1 Posteroanterior (A) and lateral (B) chest radiographs showing a small right pleural effusion.

Physical Examination and Early Clinical Findings

At admission, the patient was afebrile, alert, and cooperative, with slight respiratory symptoms at rest. Oxygen saturation measured with pulse oximetry was 95% on room air, heart rate was 78 beats/min, respiratory rate was 16 breaths/min, and blood pressure was 120/80 mm Hg. On chest examination, breath sounds were greatly reduced in the lower right hemithorax. No pallor, clubbing, or peripheral edema was observed. Chest ultrasonography (Fig. 2.2) and chest computed tomography (CT) (Fig. 2.3) confirmed right-sided pleural effusion and revealed bilateral pleural plaques.

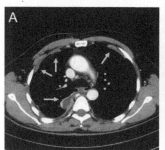
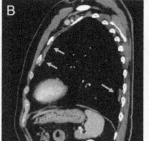
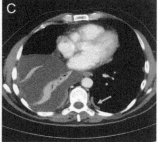

Fig. 2.2 Ultrasound images. (A) (Convex probe): right pleural effusion (*asterisk*) above the diaphragm (*arrowheads*) and atelectatic lung (*star*). (B) (Linear probe): well-defined area of echo-poor tissue (*line with arrows*) adjacent to the right lateral chest wall, corresponding to a noncalcified pleural plaque.

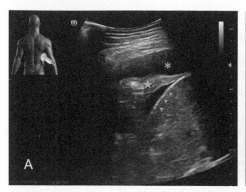
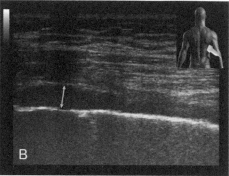

Fig. 2.3 Chest computed tomography (CT) scan. Axial (A) and sagittal (B) reconstructions showing bilateral pleural thickening and plaques (*arrows*) with rare calcifications. Axial view (C) showing right pleural effusion and pulmonary atelectasis.

Discussion Topic

Pulmonologist A

The patient has clearly been exposed to asbestos. We should understand if he has only benign pleural lesions or a malignant pleural mesothelioma.

Pulmonologist B

I would be less worried if he only had plaques. The presence of pleural effusion, although small, is more likely to be caused by malignancy, although benign asbestos pleural effusion (BAPE) is also possible.

Discussion Topic—cont'd

Pulmonologist A

I get it. You will take a look inside the pleural cavity, right?

Pulmonologist B

Exactly, medical thoracoscopy is the quickest and most effective method for obtaining a diagnosis.

Pulmonologist A

Would you have done the same if he only had pleural plaques?

Pulmonologist B

No, in the presence of pleural plaques only, I would not have proposed thoracoscopy.

Pulmonologist A

Could positron emission tomography (PET) give us additional information?

Pulmonologist B

Pleural uptake of fluorodeoxyglucose (FDG) would increase the suspicion of malignant mesothelioma. However, a negative PET result would not rule it out. So I would perform thoracoscopy even without PET.

Clinical Course

Because of the modest pleural effusion and the history of asbestos exposure, the medical team opted for diagnostic medical thoracoscopy, not preceded by thoracentesis or thoracic drainage. Thoracoscopy showed diffuse pleural plaques and nodules (Fig. 2.4). Several biopsies of the parietal pleura were performed. Histological examination revealed hyalinized collagen plaques and large areas of stromal invasion by epithelioid malignant pleural mesothelioma (MPM) with the following immunohistochemical pattern: calretinin positive, epithelial membrane antigen (EMA) positive, thyroid transcription factor 1 (TTF-1) negative, epithelial cell adhesion molecule (Ber-EP4) negative; carcinoembryonic antigen (CEA) negative (Fig. 2.5). After thoracoscopy, a drainage tube was maintained for 8 days. Subsequently talc slurry pleurodesis via chest tube was performed to reduce the risk of recurrence of pleural effusion.

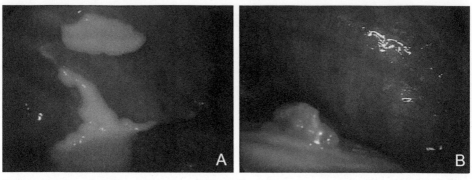

Fig. 2.4 Thoracoscopic view. (A) White regions of pleural thickening corresponding to pleural plaques. (B) Pleural nodule and diffuse pleural thickening caused by malignant proliferation.

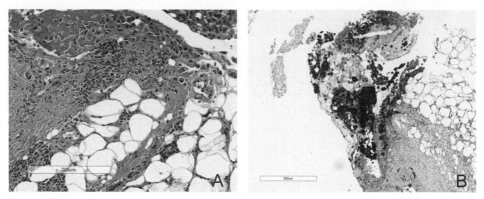

Fig. 2.5 Microscopic appearance of the malignant epithelioid mesothelioma invading fat at hematoxylin-eosin (H&E) stain (A), and immunohistochemistry stain with calretinin (B).

Discussion Topic

Pulmonologist A

Have you seen the histology report? It is an epithelioid pleural mesothelioma. What treatment options do we have?

Pulmonologist B

Probably none can significantly change the course of the disease. Even today, pleural mesothelioma is a disease with a poor prognosis despite all the efforts. Because the patient has few symptoms, I only suggest observation.

Thoracic surgeon

Because the patient has a good performance status, I propose an aggressive approach.

Discussion Topic—cont'd

Pulmonologist A

What do you mean?

Thoracic surgeon

We have at least two possible surgical options: extrapleural pneumonectomy and pleurectomy/decortication. Anyway, surgery as the only treatment is usually insufficient. It should be combined with chemotherapy and postoperative radiotherapy.

Pulmonologist B

Surgery is very invasive, and chemotherapy has many side effects! Perhaps the patient would survive a few more weeks or months. But with what quality of life? Only supportive care would be preferable.

Thoracic surgeon

I would not resign myself to merely watching the inexorable progression of the disease.

Pulmonologist A

We need to discuss the possible treatments with the patient. We must explain the risks and the extent of thoracic surgery in detail, honestly admitting that the clinical benefit is uncertain.

Recommended Therapy and Further Indications at Discharge

The patient was discharged with prescribed analgesic therapy (paracetamol). The case was discussed in a multidisciplinary team meeting. Because the patient had World Health Organization [WHO] performance status 1 (= good), surgical management (pleurectomy/decortication) was proposed. The patient was made aware of the uncertain benefit of surgery on survival and its potential impact on quality of life, and he declined surgical intervention. Thus first-line chemotherapy with pemetrexed plus cisplatin was proposed.

Follow-Up and Outcomes

The patient underwent six cycles of pemetrexed 500 mg/m^2 plus cisplatin 75 mg/m^2, administered once every 21 days. During chemotherapy, he also received folic acid (600 µg per day orally) and vitamin B$_{12}$ (1000 µg every 9 weeks, intramuscularly). Dexamethasone was also administered on the days immediately before, including, and after pemetrexed dosing to reduce the risk of severe skin rash.

The patient's disease was stable for 9 months; however, new right pleural lesions were detected subsequently, with development of increasing pain, cachexia, and progressive dyspnea. He died 3 months later as a result of a massive pulmonary embolism.

Focus On

Histological and Molecular Diagnosis of Malignant Pleural Mesothelioma

The diagnosis of malignant pleural mesothelioma (MPM) is usually determined or strongly suspected on the basis of the results of routine hematoxylin-eosin (H&E) staining. There are three major subtypes of MPM epithelioid (the most common form, about 60% of all cases), sarcomatoid (about 10% of all cases), and mixed or biphasic. Furthermore, rare subtypes include desmoplastic mesothelioma, small cell mesothelioma, and lymphohistiocytoid mesothelioma. Sarcomatoid histology, followed by mixed/biphasic histology, has a worse prognosis compared with epithelioid histology.

Immunohistochemical analyses are essential for identifying the type and particularly for distinguishing metastatic adenocarcinomas from epithelioid mesothelioma. The diagnosis of MPM is supported by the positivity of at least two markers for mesothelial differentiation and the negativity of at least two negative markers for lesions considered in the differential diagnosis.

The main markers of MPM are calretinin, Wilms tumor antigen 1 (WT-1), epithelial membrane antigen (EMA), and low-molecular-weight cytokeratins, such as CK5 and CK6.

Negative markers include Ber-EP4 (membrane marker), thyroid transcription factor 1 (TTF-1, a nuclear marker), carcinoembryonic antigen (CEA, very useful for distinguishing metastatic carcinoma, particularly of pulmonary origin, from mesothelioma), and endoplasmic reticulum (ER, commonly found in metastatic breast tumors). When the tumor has a sarcomatous component, the absence of p63 and MOC 31 (also known as epithelial specific antigen/Ep-CAM) may help distinguish it from metastases.

MPM can sometimes be difficult to distinguish from reactive mesothelial hyperplasia (RMH), a benign condition that often mimics the features of a neoplasm (high cellularity, several mitotic figures, cytological atypia, formation of papillary groups, presence of necrosis, and entrapment of mesothelial cells within fibrosis mimicking invasion).

Two new markers have recently proven useful in distinguishing benign lesions from MPM, namely, *p16*, a tumor suppressor gene, and BRCA1-associated protein 1 (BAP1). Deletion of *p16* is one of the most common cytogenetic abnormalities in MPM, found in 50% to 80% of cases. BAP1 loss can occur as a result of gene deletion, point mutations, or other indirect mechanisms and is found in 15% to 60% of cases. Both *p16* deletion and BAP1 loss have a specificity of 100% for MPM.

Focus On

Imaging Techniques in the Diagnosis of Malignant Pleural Mesothelioma

Chest radiography is historically the first step in the diagnosis of MPM. It allows detecting its main manifestation (i.e., pleural effusion and pleural thickening or masses).

Chest ultrasonography is being increasingly used to visualize pleural effusion and pleural thickening or nodules and to identify lung lesions with at least a small degree of contact with the pleura. It also helps guide diagnostic procedures such as thoracentesis, needle aspiration, and core biopsies.

Computed tomography (CT), preferably with contrast medium, allows for better definition of such alterations and to choose the best diagnostic approach. Thickening of the mediastinal pleura and the interlobar pleura is highly suggestive of malignancy.

Positron emission tomography (PET) can provide useful information regarding functional aspects. Maximum standard uptake values (SUV_{max}) greater than 2.0 usually allow for differentiation of malignant pleural disease from benign pleural disease and has a sensitivity of about 95% but is poorly specific for MPM. It should be noted, however, that PET results can be markedly abnormal after pleurodesis.

Small-volume tumors with a low proliferative index (e.g., early-stage epithelioid mesothelioma) are among the causes of false-negative PET findings.

The combination of PET findings and the morphological data from CT scan (PET-CT) is particularly useful for preoperative staging of MPM, for evaluating treatment response, and for detecting possible recurrence.

Focus On

Management of Malignant Pleural Mesothelioma

MPM is a disease with a poor prognosis and limited therapeutic options. Each patient with MPM should be evaluated by an expert multidisciplinary team. The proposed treatment should depend on the extent of disease, the patient's general condition (age, performance status, cardiopulmonary function, comorbidities), and patient preference for aggressive potentially curative treatment or palliative treatment.

MPM is considered resectable if it is restricted to a single location and has not spread to the lymph nodes or other organs and tissues. The two main surgical approaches for MPM are extrapleural pneumonectomy (EPP), in which the lung is removed en bloc, along with the parietal pericardium, parietal pleura, and diaphragmatic pleura; and extended pleurectomy/decortication (EPD), in which the lung is left intact. Both EPP and EPD are associated with significant morbidity and mortality, although a better outcome has been observed in centers with high expertise. A multimodal approach with combination of surgery, radiotherapy, and chemotherapy has also been proposed. That being said, there are no randomized trials suggesting improved mortality rates with surgery, and current guidelines suggest that surgery for mesothelioma should only be performed in the setting of clinical trials.

Chemotherapy usually consists of a platinum-based agent, such as cisplatin, often combined with a folate antimetabolite, such as pemetrexed. Immunotherapy has been recently proposed as a further possible therapeutic choice for MPM.

Patient-centered outcomes, such as acceptable quality of life, relief of dyspnea, and shorter time in the hospital should be the primary goals of care in these patients.

LEARNING POINTS

- Asbestos exposure is the main risk factor for MPM and is responsible for at least 85% of cases.
- The latency period between the first asbestos exposure and the development of MPM is very long, usually 30 to 40 years.
- The finding of pleural plaques is an indicator of previous exposure to asbestos fibers and not a marker of malignancy.
- The gold standard to diagnose MPM is histological examination of adequate pleural biopsy specimens obtained in the context of proper clinical, radiological, and surgical findings.
- Only a few MPMs exfoliate tumor cells; thus effusion cytology is rarely diagnostic.
- Surgical approaches alone to treat MPM offer poor benefit in terms of survival and symptom relief and have high operative mortality and recurrence rate.

Further Reading

1. Woolhouse I, Bishop L, Darlison L, et al. BTS guideline for the investigation and management of malignant pleural mesothelioma. *BMJ Open Respir Res.* 2018;5(1):e000266.
2. Husain AN, Colby TV, Ordo'nez NG, et al. Guidelines for pathologic diagnosis of malignant mesothelioma. 2017 update of the consensus statement from the International Mesothelioma Interest Group. *Arch Pathol Lab Med.* 2018;142(1):89–108.
3. Porcel JM, Hernández P, Martínez-Alonso M, et al. Accuracy of fluorodeoxyglucose-PET imaging for differentiating benign from malignant pleural effusions: a meta-analysis. *Chest.* 2015;147:502.
4. Pairon JC, Laurent F, Rinaldo M, et al. Pleural plaques and the risk of pleural mesothelioma. *J Natl Cancer Inst.* 2013;105:293.
5. American Thoracic Society. Diagnosis and initial management of nonmalignant diseases related to asbestos. *Am J Respir Crit Care Med.* 2004;170:691.
6. de Fonseka D, Underwood W, Stadon L, et al. Randomised controlled trial to compare the diagnostic yield of positron emission tomography CT (PET-CT) TARGETed pleural biopsy versus CT-guided pleural biopsy in suspected pleural malignancy (TARGET trial). *BMJ Open Respir Res.* 2018;5(1):e000270.

7. Xu LL, Yang Y, Wang Z, et al. Malignant pleural mesothelioma: diagnostic value of medical thoracoscopy and long-term prognostic analysis. *BMC Pulm Med.* 2018;18(1):56.
8. Katzman D, Sterman DH. Updates in the diagnosis and treatment of malignant pleural mesothelioma. *Curr Opin Pulm Med.* 2018;24(4):319–326.
9. Kindler HL, Ismaila N, Armato SG, 3rd, et al. Treatment of malignant pleural mesothelioma: American Society of Clinical Oncology Clinical Practice Guideline. *J Clin Oncol.* 2018;36(13):1343–1373.
10. Sharif S, Zahid I, Routledge T, Scarci M. Extrapleural pneumonectomy or supportive care: treatment of malignant pleural mesothelioma. *Interact Cardiovasc Thorac Surg.* 2011;12(6):1040–1045.
11. Bonomi M, De Filippis C, Lopci E, et al. Clinical staging of malignant pleural mesothelioma: current perspectives. *Lung Cancer (Auckl).* 2017;8:127–139.
12. Berzenji L, Van Schil P. Multimodality treatment of malignant pleural mesothelioma. *Res.* 2018;7:F1000.
13. Liu J, Liao X, Gu Y, et al. Role of p16 deletion and BAP1 loss in the diagnosis of malignant mesothelioma. *J Thorac Dis.* 2018;10(9):5522–5530.
14. Rintoul RC, Ritchie AJ, Edwards JG, et al. Efficacy and cost of video-assisted thoracoscopic partial pleurectomy versus talc pleurodesis in patients with malignant pleural mesothelioma (MesoVATS): an open-label, randomised, controlled trial. *Lancet.* 2014;384(9948):1118–1127.
15. Zalcman G, Mazieres J, Margery J, et al. Bevacizumab for newly diagnosed pleural mesothelioma in the Mesothelioma Avastin Cisplatin Pemetrexed Study (MAPS): a randomised, controlled, open-label, phase 3 trial [published correction appears in Lancet. 2016 Apr 2;387(10026):e24]. *Lancet.* 2016;387(10026):1405–1414.
16. Treasure T, Lang-Lazdunski L, Waller D, et al. Extra-pleural pneumonectomy versus no extra-pleural pneumonectomy for patients with malignant pleural mesothelioma: clinical outcomes of the Mesothelioma and Radical Surgery (MARS) randomised feasibility study. *Lancet Oncol.* 2011;12(8):763–772.

CHAPTER 3

Malignant Pleural Effusion in Metastatic Pulmonary Adenocarcinoma Complicated by Pulmonary Embolism

Claudio Sorino ■ David Feller-Kopman ■ Giampietro Marchetti ■ Mario Spatafora

History of Present Illness

A 71-year-old woman had been suffering for about 1 month from weakness, daytime sleepiness, loss of appetite with weight loss of 2 kg, low-grade fever (37.8° C [104° F]), diffuse chest pain, exertional dyspnea, and dry cough.

The general practitioner ordered chest radiography, which showed dense opacity in the right upper pulmonary field, and antibiotic therapy (levofloxacin 500 mg daily for 6 days, followed by amoxicillin/clavulanic acid 1000 mg twice a day for 7 days). Because of persisting fever and worsening dyspnea, the patient went to the emergency room.

Past Medical History

The patient was a lifetime nonsmoker. The most significant events in her medical history were arterial hypertension, mild dyslipidemia, and angioplasty with stenting of the left main coronary artery 4 years ago. She was currently under therapy with bisoprolol 1.25 mg/day, ramipril 2.5 mg/day, amlodipine 5 mg/day, acetylsalicylic acid 100 mg/day, and atorvastatin 20 mg/day.

Physical Examination and Early Clinical Findings

Blood tests showed mild leukocytosis (white blood cell [WBC] count 10,130/mm³) and increased inflammatory markers (C-reactive protein [CRP] 66.2 mg/L, normal values < 10 mg/L) and lactate dehydrogenase (LDH; 2359 units/L, normal values < 618 units/L).

Chest radiography confirmed the presence of opacity in the posterior region of the right upper lobe and homolateral basal pleural effusion with fissure involvement (Fig. 3.1).

Clinical Course

The patient underwent chest/abdominal CT before and after administration of contrast medium (Figs. 3.2 and 3.3). The right lung had a reduced volume compared with the contralateral lung. In the dorsal segment of the right upper lobe, there was a solid hyperdense round lesion with irregular margins, about 4 cm in diameter, surrounded by thickened interlobular septa. The mass crossed the major fissure, also involving the apex of the right lower lobe. On the same side, the CT scan showed pleural effusion, with maximum thickness of about 3 cm, and dysventilation of

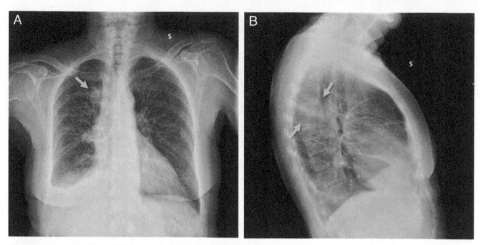

Fig. 3.1   Posteroanterior (A) and lateral (B) chest radiograph obtained upon admission, showing lung opacity in the posterior region of the right upper lobe (*arrows*). Homolateral basal pleural effusion with fissure involvement is also visible.

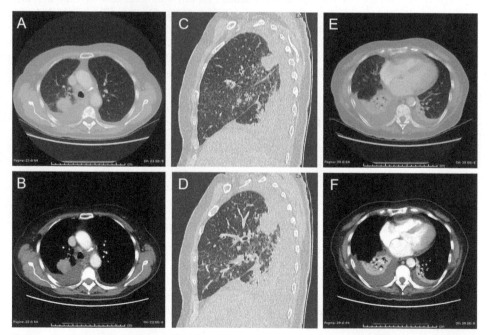

Fig. 3.2   Chest computed tomography (CT) images showing a solid, round lesion in the dorsal segment of the right upper lobe. (A, B) Axial scans of lung and mediastinum window. (C, D) Sagittal scans. (E, F) Bilateral pleural effusion with dysventilation of the adjacent lower pulmonary lobes.

the posterior segment of the right lower lobe. A small pleural effusion (maximum thickness of about 15 mm) was also present on the left side. Several enlarged lymph nodes, with a diameter of about 15 mm, were detected in paratracheal sites. The liver was widely altered by multiple, small, hypodense lesions, some with peripheral enhancement (target or "bull's eye" lesions).

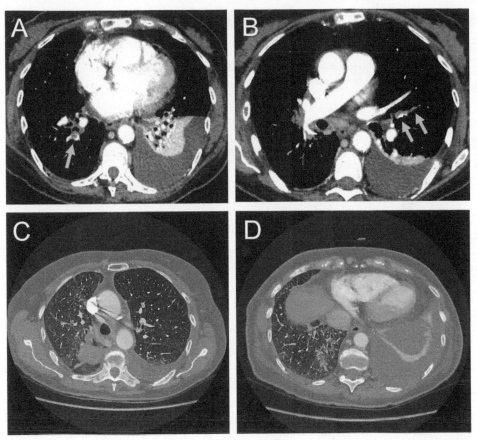

Fig. 3.3 Computed tomography pulmonary angiography (CTPA), performed for acute worsening of symptoms despite right thoracentesis. (A, B) Some of the bilateral perfusion defects caused by pulmonary embolism are evident (*arrows*). (C) The lung cancer is clearly recognizable in the right upper lobe. The mass crossed the major fissure, also involving the apex of the right lower lobe. (D) The left pleural effusion increased, whereas the right pleural effusion had been drained.

Discussion Topic

Pulmonologist

I just saw the computed tomography (CT) scans of the chest and abdomen. No good news for the patient: she has a right lung cancer with lymph node and hepatic involvement.

Pulmonologist B

The very high lactate dehydrogenase (LDH) value is a negative prognostic biomarker. What can we do now?

Continued

Discussion Topic—cont'd

Pulmonologist A

How about thoracoscopy? It could be useful for diagnosis and also could allow concomitant pleurodesis.

Pulmonologist B

I would start with less invasive procedures: bronchoscopy and thoracentesis. If we do not get a histological diagnosis, transthoracic needle biopsy could be a further option.

Pulmonologist A

We must involve the patient in this decision; she has to be informed about the results of the CT scan, and then we can discuss the possible diagnostic procedures with her.

Pulmonologist B

The patient is taking low-dose aspirin for coronary artery disease. Should it be discontinued?

Pulmonologist A

It could be continued if the patient will be undergoing only thoracentesis. However, because we'll probably need to perform bronchial biopsy or transthoracic needle biopsy, I suggest stopping it.

Pulmonologist B

We should also look for bone and brain metastases. Staging should be completed with bone scintigraphy and brain CT.

After obtaining informed consent from the patient, right thoracentesis was performed, resulting in drainage of 500 mL of pleural fluid. Bronchoscopy was scheduled for the next day. However, during the night, the patient experienced severe worsening of dyspnea, and severe hypoxemic respiratory failure occurred. Blood tests showed a rise in WBC (16,830/mm^3) and CRP (285.8 mg/L); intravenous antibiotic therapy with imipenem/cilastatin (500/500 mg four times daily) and linezolid (600 mg two times daily) was started. Because of a significant increase in d-dimer (6716 ng/mL), chest CT angiography was performed, and it showed multiple filling defects on the arterial segmental branches in the left upper lobe and the right lower lobe. Hence, a diagnosis of diffuse pulmonary embolism (PE) was made; interestingly, although the right pleural effusion had almost disappeared, a significant amount of left pleural effusion had developed (see Fig. 3.3). Echocardiography showed an increase in estimated pulmonary artery systolic pressure (PASP; 40 mm Hg), whereas color Doppler ultrasonography ruled out deep venous thrombosis (DVT) in the lower limbs. Subcutaneous enoxaparin 100 units/kg two times daily was promptly started.

Cytology of the pleural fluid yielded a positive result for cancer cells, and morphology and immune-cytochemical profile were suggestive of pleural involvement by lung adenocarcinoma (tumor cells positive for epithelial cell adhesion molecule [Ber-EP4], thyroid transcription factor 1 [TTF-1], and napsin). However, the low proportion of cancer cells in the pleural effusion did not allow for testing for epidermal growth factor receptor *(EGFR)* gene abnormalities, anaplastic lymphoma kinase (ALK) rearrangements, or programmed death ligand 1 (PD-L1) expression.

CT of the brain showed several hyperdense round lesions suggestive of cerebral metastases from the lung cancer. Technetium-99m methylene diphosphonate (Tc-99m MDP) bone scintigraphy demonstrated multiple tracer uptakes resulting from widespread metastatic bone disease (skull, sternum, scapulae, ribs, spine, pelvis, left and right humeri, femurs, and fibulae).

Discussion Topic

Pulmonologist A

The patient's clinical condition will not allow for administration of active chemotherapy treatments. She has asthenia, dyspnea even with minimal effort, and inability to carry on any self-care, and she is confined to bed or chair for most of her waking hours. Her Eastern Cooperative Oncology Group (ECOG) performance status score is 4.

Pulmonologist B

However, it is worth checking if the patient can be a candidate for targeted therapy or immunotherapy. The prevalence of *EGFR* gene abnormalities is higher among female never-smokers.

Pulmonologist C

We could perform transthoracic needle biopsy of the lung mass. The sample should allow search for epidermal growth factor receptor *(EGFR)* mutations, anaplastic lymphoma kinase *(ALK)* gene rearrangement, and expression of programmed death ligand 1 (PD-L1) in malignant cells.

Pulmonologist B

Alternatively, we could try to obtain a tissue sample via needle biopsy of a supraclavicular lymph node. The procedure is safer than transthoracic needle biopsy.

Pulmonologist A

I agree. The patient no longer takes aspirin, but she is on anticoagulant therapy. We should stop it before the needle biopsy, right?

Pulmonologist C

Yes, we should stop low-molecular-weight heparin (LMWH) administration only 12 hours before biopsy.

Discussion Topic

Pulmonologist A

Do you think evacuating the left pleural effusion can alleviate the patient's dyspnea?

Pulmonologist B

It's possible. However, several other factors may contribute to her breathlessness: lung cancer, pulmonary embolism with acute pulmonary hypertension, probably also respiratory infection, and congestive heart failure.

Pulmonologist C

We could place a left chest tube while anticoagulant therapy is suspended. This would allow a subsequent talc slurry pleurodesis.

Pulmonologist B

I don't agree. I usually perform pleurodesis if I am certain that the pleural effusion is malignant. In our patient, the left pleural effusion could be related to an excess of fluids. Indeed, the primary tumor is located in the opposite right lung, and the inferior vena cava appears slightly dilated on ultrasonography. I would increase diuretic therapy.

Pulmonologist A

I would suggest starting with thoracentesis. It would allow us to analyze the pleural effusion and verify if the patient has any relief of symptoms. If necessary, it can be repeated later.

The patient underwent ultrasound-guided needle biopsy of a left supraclavicular lymph node. Enoxaparin administration had been suspended 12 hours before the procedure and was resumed 12 hours later. At the same time, left thoracentesis was performed to reduce dyspnea, and approximately 1200 mL of the pleural effusion was evacuated. Because of the widespread pain and worsening dyspnea, administration of morphine was started. Histology of the lymph node confirmed metastatic tissue from pulmonary adenocarcinoma. No mutation of the *EGFR* gene or rearrangements of ALK and reactive oxygen species 1 (ROS1) were found. Moreover, the tumor cells had low PD-L1 expression. These results precluded initiation of targeted therapy or immunotherapy. The patient was discharged and sent for best supportive care in a hospice facility, where she continued to receive high-flow oxygen and opioid (fentanyl) at progressively higher doses. No further evacuation of pleural fluid was necessary. Death occurred 20 days later.

Focus On

Molecular Testing of Advanced Non–Small Cell Lung Cancer

Some genetic mutations have been shown to play a key role in the progression of non–small cell lung cancer (NSCLC), mainly lung adenocarcinoma, to metastatic disease. When a lung adenocarcinoma or a mixed lung cancer with an adenocarcinoma component is diagnosed, molecular testing is strongly recommended to select patients eligible for therapies directed at specific genetic alterations ("targeted therapies").

Focus On—cont'd

The *EGFR* (epidermal growth factor receptor) gene is mutated in 20% to 40% of patients with lung adenocarcinoma. *EGFR* mutation frequency is higher among women, never-smokers, and Southeast Asians. *EGFR* inhibitors (erlotinib, gefitinib, and afatinib) are the targeted cancer therapies available for *EGFR* mutations.

ALK (anaplastic lymphoma kinase) gene rearrangement occurs in 5% to 7% of lung adenocarcinomas. This mutation is strongly associated with a history of never or light smoking (< 10 pack-years). *ALK* rearrangement has been reported in squamous cell carcinoma, but this is rare.

ROS1 (reactive oxygen species 1) gene rearrangement is found in 1% to 2% of lung adenocarcinomas, more commonly in light smokers (< 10 pack-years) and/or never-smokers.

Crizotinib is a multitarget molecule, approved for the treatment of both *ALK* and *ROS1* gene rearrangement.

KRAS (Kirsten rat sarcoma) gene mutation is found in 20% to 30% of lung adenocarcinomas, but no targeted therapy for this mutation is currently available in clinical practice.

The expression of *PD-L1* (programmed death ligand 1) on lung adenocarcinomas or other solid tumors has been shown to predict response to checkpoint inhibitors (e.g., pembrolizumab, nivolumab, atezolizumab, and others) that improve the antitumor capacity of the immune system.

Focus On

Management of Anticoagulant and Antiplatelet Agents in Adults Undergoing Percutaneous Interventions

Before performing a percutaneous procedure in a patient receiving antithrombotic therapy, the risk of bleeding with continued treatment and the risk of thrombosis resulting from suspension of the therapy should be weighed against each other.

Usually thoracentesis is considered to have a low risk of bleeding, whereas transthoracic needle biopsy, chest tube insertion, and thoracoscopy may involve a moderate or high risk (depending on other patient features, such as renal failure).

Bridging anticoagulation therapy with heparin can minimize thrombotic events in high-risk patients, such as those who have experienced recent stroke, thromboembolic event, coronary stent placement, mechanical heart valve, or prior venous thromboembolism during interruption of chronic anticoagulation therapy.

Aspirin therapy should be discontinued only if surgical hemostasis is predicted to be difficult. In patients receiving mandatory dual antiplatelet therapy, the less invasive procedure should be performed, and if possible, it should be postponed until at least one drug can be temporarily suspended.

Table 3.1 shows a simplified schematic for determining the optimal timing for withdrawal of anticoagulant or antiplatelet drugs before chest percutaneous procedures. If hemostasis is maintained, resumption of the antiplatelet drugs can begin immediately after the procedure. Anticoagulants are usually reintroduced after 12 to 24 hours.

Focus On

Venous Thromboembolism in Cancer: Early Diagnostic and Therapeutic Approach

Venous thromboembolism (VTE) is a condition in which blood clots form in the deep vein of the legs or arms (deep venous thrombosis [DVT]), may break free, and reach the right heart and then the lungs (pulmonary embolism [PE]). Cancer is a well-recognized predisposing factor for VTE.

As an immediately life-threatening condition, PE requires emergent diagnostic evaluation (usually with computed tomography pulmonary angiography [CTPA] or ventilation/perfusion lung scintigraphy) and treatment.

When PE is suspected or diagnosed, lower limb compression ultrasonography (CUS) is recommended to evaluate for DVT. In addition, echocardiography is useful because PE may cause right ventricle pressure overload and dysfunction.

Continued

Focus On—cont'd

Rescue thrombolytic therapy is recommended for patients experiencing hemodynamic deterioration. For most cases of PE without hemodynamic compromise, anticoagulant therapy is recommended.

Subcutaneous low-molecular-weight heparin (LMWH) or fondaparinux can significantly decrease the risk of VTE recurrence, with lower risk of major bleeding compared with vitamin K antagonists (VKAs). Thus LMWH or fondaparinux has long been considered the standard of care. An equally rapid anticoagulant effect can also be achieved with a non–vitamin K antagonist oral anticoagulant (NOAC). NOACs could make the treatment easier because of their oral administration in fixed-dose regimens. As a consequence, they are currently the first choice in eligible patients. Edoxaban and rivaroxaban should also be considered as alternatives to LMWH in patients with malignancy. Caution should be exercised in patients with gastrointestinal cancer because of the increased bleeding risk.

The insertion of a venous filter is indicated in VTE when anticoagulation is impossible because of hemorrhage or a high bleeding risk.

Anticoagulants should be continued indefinitely unless, after proper treatment, there is evidence that the patient is free of cancer.

TABLE 3.1 ■ **Suggested Intervals Between the Suspension of Anticoagulant or Antiplatelet Agents and a Thoracic Percutaneous Procedure**

Agent	Interval Between Last Dose and Procedure
Warfarin	Until international normalized ratio (INR) < 1.5, usually 3–6 days
Unfractionated heparin	Intravenous: 2–6 hours subcutaneous: 12–24 hours
Low-molecular-weight heparin (LMWH; e.g., enoxaparin)	12 hours
Fondaparinux	36–48 hours
Rivaroxaban	Normal renal function: ≥ 1 days Creatinine clearance (CrCl): 60–90 mL/min, 2 days CrCl: 30–59 mL/min, 3 days CrCl: 15–29 mL/min, 4 days
Dabigatran	CrCl: ≥ 50 mL/min, 1–2 day CrCl: <50 mL/min, 3–5 days
Apixaban	CrCl: – 60 mL/min, 1–2 days CrCl: 50–59 mL/min, 3 days CrCl: <30–49 mL/min, 5 days
Desirudin	2 hours
Aspirin	Low or moderate risk: None High risk: 5 days
Clopidogrel	5 days
Ticagrelor	5 days
Prasugrel	5–7 days
Ticlopidine	10–14 days

LEARNING POINTS

- Histological definition of lung cancer should include tests to verify the feasibility of targeted therapy or immunotherapy.
- Cytology samples (mainly cell blocks) can be used to reliably detect EGFR mutations and ALK rearrangements.
- Thoracic percutaneous procedures with a low bleeding risk can be safely performed without suspension of low-dose aspirin.
- For patients with pulmonary embolism (PE) and cancer, low-molecular-weight heparin (LMWH) should be considered for the first 6 months over vitamin K antagonists (VKAs).
- Edoxaban or rivaroxaban are valid alternatives to LMWH in patients with PE and malignancy other than gastrointestinal cancer.
- For patients with PE and cancer, extended anticoagulation should be performed for an indefinite period until the cancer is cured or death occurs.

Further Reading

1. Joshi A, Pande N, Noronha V, et al. ROS1 mutation non-small cell lung cancer-access to optimal treatment and outcomes. *Ecancermedicalscience*. 2019;13:900.
2. Palumbo G, Carillio G, Manzo A, et al. Pembrolizumab in lung cancer: current evidence and future perspectives. *Future Oncol*. 2019;15(29):3327–3336.
3. Liu X, Wang P, Zhang C, Ma Z. Epidermal growth factor receptor (EGFR): a rising star in the era of precision medicine of lung cancer. *Oncotarget*. 2017;8(30):50209–50220.
4. Kennedy SA, Milovanovic L, Midia M. Major bleeding after percutaneous image-guided biopsies: frequency, predictors, and periprocedural management. *Semin Intervent Radiol*. 2015;32:26–33.
5. Konstantinides SV, Meyer G, Becattini C, et al.; ESC Scientific Document Group. 2019 ESC guidelines for the diagnosis and management of acute pulmonary embolism developed in collaboration with the European Respiratory Society (ERS): the Task Force for the diagnosis and management of acute pulmonary embolism of the European Society of Cardiology (ESC). *Eur Heart J*. 2020;41(4):543–603.
6. Kazandjian D, Gong Y, Keegan P, et al. Prognostic value of the lung immune prognostic index for patients treated for metastatic non-small cell lung cancer. *JAMA Oncol*. 2019;5(10):1481–1485.
7. Boeckx B, Shahi RB, Smeets D, et al. The genomic landscape of nonsmall cell lung carcinoma in never smokers. *Int J Cancer*. 2020;146(11):3207–3218.

CHAPTER 4

Squamous Cell Lung Cancer Complicating a Tuberculous Fibrothorax

Giampietro Marchetti ▪ Claudio Sorino ▪ David Feller-Kopman
▪ Stefano Elia

History of Present Illness

An 82-year-old man presented to the outpatient pulmonary clinic because in the past 4 weeks he had worsening breathlessness and low-grade fever. He also had a mild, chronic, cough without sputum and had a weight loss of about 3 kg in 3 months. Chest radiography, ordered by his general practitioner, revealed bilateral calcified pleural plaques, more on the right than on the left, and further opacity in the right mid-zone (Fig. 4.1).

Past Medical History

The patient had never smoked and had worked as a truck driver. When he was 25 years old, he had been diagnosed with pulmonary tuberculosis and had undergone artificial right pneumothorax. His medical history also included arterial hypertension and prostatic hypertrophy.

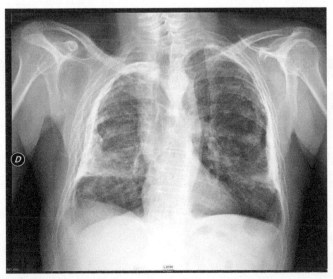

Fig. 4.1 Posteroanterior chest radiograph showing bilateral pleural thickening, with calcific plaques caused by fibrothorax. Additional opacity in the right mid-zone and volume loss of the right thorax, with mild mediastinal shift to the right, are also evident.

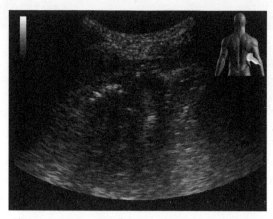

Fig. 4.2 Chest ultrasound showing layers of the thorax and the interface between the lung and the pleura, which are difficult to distinguish because of fibrothorax. A hypogenic area compatible with fluid collection is also noticeable.

Physical Examination and Early Clinical Findings

The patient was hemodynamically stable, with oxygen saturation of 93% in room air and body temperature of 37.2° C [98.9° F]. Physical examination revealed widely reduced breath sounds, mainly on the right side, and fine crackles at the lower zones. Recent blood tests had shown slight leukocytosis (white blood cell [WBC] count: 12,500 cells/μL, with 59.6% neutrophils and 31.8% lymphocytes) and a small increase in the inflammation indices (C-reactive protein [CRP]: 28 mg/L, normal values < 5 mg/L). No results of previous chest computed tomography (CT) or x-ray were available. Chest ultrasonography (Fig. 4.2) showed narrowed intercostal spaces, whereas the pleural line and the gliding sign were difficult to observe. At the right base, an anechoic area compatible with fluid collection was appreciated.

Chest CT showed a round mass with smooth margins and a nonhomogeneous fluid content, located in the posterior region of the right lower lobe, contiguous with the calcified fibrothorax (Figs. 4.3, A–C).

Discussion Topic

Pulmonologist A

Do you think the lesion in the lower right lobe is of pulmonary or pleural origin?

Radiologist

This is not easy to answer. It is contiguous with the pleural calcifications; however, it seems to be centered in the lung, and I don't recognize the pleura around it. Moreover, its angles with the chest wall are not clearly obtuse as I would expect if the origin was pleural.

Pulmonologist B

Chest computed tomography (CT) also suggests a central area of colliquation, probably caused by necrosis.

Discussion Topic—cont'd

Pulmonologist A

We should consider chronic tuberculous empyema and lung cancer in the differential diagnosis. I believe that positron emission tomography (PET) can provide useful information on local metabolic activity and other possible localizations.

Pulmonologist B

I would perform an ultrasound-guided puncture to evaluate the characteristics of the liquid and the presence of active tuberculosis.

Pulmonologist A

I'm afraid that pricking a tuberculous bag can be dangerous. It could cause a pleurocutaneous fistula. Moreover, passage of a needle through the calcified layer of fibrothorax is not easy at all. The patient has a fever. Why don't we start an ex juvantibus therapy for *Mycobacterium tuberculosis*?

Pulmonologist B

I don't like the idea. We need to know what the patient actually has.

Pulmonologist A

We should also search for mycobacteria in other samples: sputum, bronchial lavage, urine, gastric juice …

The patient was admitted for further investigations. Thoracic ultrasonography allowed for identification of a space among the pleural calcifications, through which a 14-gauge needle was introduced until it reached the fluid collection. Passage of the needle through the thickened and calcified pleura was difficult. Only 5 mL of odorless, beige-colored liquid was extracted. In this sample, microscopic examination for acid-fast bacilli (AFB) yielded negative results, as did polymerase chain reaction (PCR) amplification of relevant DNA sequences of *Mycobacterium tuberculosis*. Sputum and urine smear microscopy results were also negative for AFB.

Whole-body ^{18}fluorodeoxyglucose (FDG) positron emission tomography (PET) was performed (Fig. 4.4). The lesion in the right lower lobe showed intense uptake in its peripheral part, with a maximum standard uptake value (SUV_{max}) of 6. No abnormal accumulation of the ^{18}FDG was found in other parts of the body.

It was determined that the patient's ECOG Performance Status was 2 and the Karnofsky Performance Status 50% (i.e., he was able to care for himself but unable to perform most work-related activities).

Discussion Topic

Pulmonologist A

In light of the results obtained, malignancy is the most likely diagnosis.

Continued

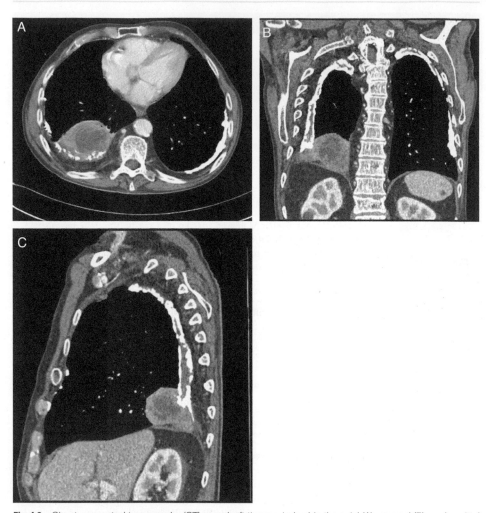

Fig. 4.3 Chest computed tomography (CT) scan (soft tissue window) in the axial (A), coronal (B), and sagittal (C) planes. Diffuse, sheet-like pleural calcification, caused by calcified fibrothorax, and volume loss of the right lung are evident. A round mass with smooth margins and nonhomogeneous fluid content is present in the posterior region of the right lower lobe.

Discussion Topic—cont'd

Pulmonologist B

If so, the necrotic area suggests a fast-growing cancer causing poor blood supply.

Pulmonologist A

Biopsy for histological examination is necessary to confirm this.

Discussion Topic—cont'd

Pulmonologist B

Before subjecting the patient to further invasive procedures, it is important to know the potential therapeutic perspectives. Is surgery possible?

Thoracic surgeon

The position of the lesion and the presence of extensive fibrothorax could require a long procedure and perhaps pneumonectomy. The patient is very old, so surgery may pose a high risk of death. A careful evaluation of the patient's performance status and measurement of lung function could allow for more precise evaluation of the risk.

Pulmonologist B

What about chemotherapy?

Oncologist

There is no evidence of distant metastasis. Because the disease appears to be confined to the lung, we can consider stereotactic radiotherapy.

Radiotherapist

Stereotactic radiotherapy is a well-established treatment option for early-stage non–small cell lung cancer less than 5 cm in size. There is limited information with regard to larger tumors. However, we have no other therapeutic options in this case.

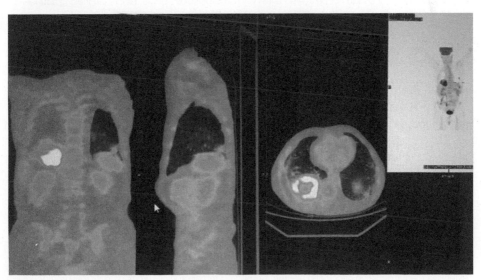

Fig. 4.4 ^{18}Fluorodeoxyglucose (FDG) positron emission tomography (PET) scan showing a peripheral uptake in the pulmonary mass of the right lower lobe.

Pulmonary function test showed a restrictive defect with forced expiratory volume in 1 second (FEV1) of 1.68 L (67.6%), forced vital capacity (FVC) of 2.33 L (69.8%), and total lung capacity (TLC) of 3.28 L (71.4%).

The radiologist performed CT-guided percutaneous biopsy of the lesion in the right lower lobe. No pneumothorax was evident after the maneuver. Results of the histological examination of the specimen led to the diagnosis of squamous cell carcinoma.

The thoracic surgeon explained the risks of surgery, and the patient chose stereotactic body radiation therapy (SBRT).

Follow-Up

The patient underwent SBRT. He received 60 Gy in three fractions (20 Gy per fraction; one every 72 hours). The lung lesion was observed to be relatively stable on chest CT scans obtained after 6 and 12 months. However, restaging at 12 months showed the appearance of brain and bone metastases.

Focus On

Late Sequelae and Complications of Tuberculosis

Residual pulmonary and extrapulmonary lesions may persist even after successful treatment of tuberculosis. These include:
- Parenchymal lesions (tuberculoma, thin-walled cavity, cicatrization, calcification, end-stage lung destruction, aspergilloma, and bronchogenic carcinoma)
- Airway lesions (bronchiectasis, tracheobronchial stenosis, and broncholithiasis)
- Vascular lesions (pulmonary or bronchial arteritis and thrombosis, bronchial artery dilatation, and Rasmussen aneurysm)
- Mediastinal lesions (lymph node calcification and extranodal extension, esophagomediastinal or esophagobronchial fistula, constrictive pericarditis, mediastinitis)
- Pleural lesions (chronic empyema, pleural thickening, fibrothorax, bronchopleural fistula, pneumothorax)
- Chest wall lesions (rib tuberculosis, tuberculous spondylitis, and malignancy associated with chronic empyema)

Sequelae can provoke symptoms even without active tuberculosis (e.g., hemoptysis, dyspnea, chronic respiratory failure) but should not be treated again with antituberculosis drugs. Before diagnosing a tuberculous sequela, it is necessary to exclude the presence of bacilli in sputum or bronchial aspirate.

Indeed, after clinical resolution of pulmonary tuberculosis, bacilli can remain alive within calcified tuberculous scars, and they can cause active tuberculosis even after several years, especially if immunosuppression occurs.

Focus On

Malignancy Associated With Chronic Empyema and Fibrothorax

Chronic empyema and fibrothorax can rarely be complicated by nonepithelial or epithelial tumors. The most frequent histopathological diagnoses are malignant lymphoma and squamous cell carcinoma. Malignancy usually develops decades after the onset of empyema or fibrothorax. Longstanding chronic inflammation inside lesions is believed to promote the neoplastic transformation.

Squamous cells could originate from the skin epithelium and reach the pleural cavity through a pleurocutaneous fistula. It is also possible that squamous metaplasia, a preneoplastic change of the bronchial epithelium, develops through a bronchopleural fistula. In cases without any those fistulas, squamous cell carcinoma might arise from the skin fragments that could enter the pleural space during pleural procedures such as thoracentesis or more commonly from squamous metaplasia of mesothelial cells.

Radiographic findings that suggest malignancy include increased chest opacity, soft tissue bulging and blurring of fat planes in the chest walls, bone destruction near the empyema or the fibrothorax, and extensive medial deviation of calcified pleurae. Computed tomography (CT) can demonstrate an abnormal mass with soft tissue attenuation, usually with contrast enhancement. Biopsy is required because clinical differentiation between malignancy and infection is often difficult.

Focus On

How to Distinguish Pleural and Extrapleural Lesions From Peripheral Pulmonary Lesions

On conventional chest radiography, a peripheral lung lesion can be difficult to distinguish from a pleural or extrapleural lesion. Computed tomography (CT) is, by far, more accurate than chest radiography. The shape and margins of the lesion may help in this evaluation (Fig. 4.5). A lung mass tends to have acute angles against adjacent pleural surfaces, whereas pleural lesions usually form obtuse, straight, or acute angles, but with tapering connecting angles. Unlike lung masses, pleural lesions appear with their maximum diameter abutting the pleural surface. Extrapleural lesions can infiltrate chest wall muscles and erode the ribs. They can also extend into the lung. In this case, they displace both pleural layers and usually have an appearance similar to the pleural ones. Despite all of the mentioned differences, some overlap exists in the cross-sectional appearance of peripheral lesions. For instance, some pleural lesions originating from the visceral pleura can be pedunculated and may be confused with lung parenchymal lesions. Conversely, a large malignant parenchymal lesion may infiltrate the pleural layers and form an obtuse angle with the chest wall, thus mimicking a pleural lesion. Attenuation coefficients also help character-ize the nature of a lesion on CT. A potential confounding factor is the presence of fluid within a lesion. This could result from colliquation of a lung mass or from liquid filling a pre-existing cavity, such as a bulla. Its appearance may resemble loculated pleural effusion. Chest ultrasonography can help differentiate pleural diseases from peripheral pulmonary lesions. A peripheral lung tumor appears as a homogeneous, well-defined mass that is usually hypoechoic and usually has a pos-terior acoustic enhancement. Moreover, ultrasonography is useful to assess chest wall invasion of tumors, with a slightly higher sensitivity, but a slight lower specificity, compared with CT. High-resolution linear ultrasound probes are best suited for this purpose. If ultrasonography shows the mass breaching the pleura and losing its movement with respiration, the tumor has extended beyond the pariotal pleura into the chest wall.

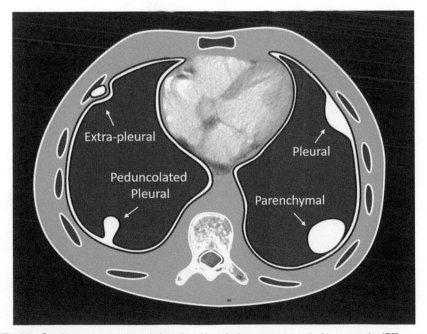

Fig. 4.5 Graphic representation of pleural and lung lesions on a computed tomography (CT) scan.

LEARNING POINTS

- Thoracic malignancies may be a rare long-term sequelae of tuberculosis, especially when chronic empyema or fibrothorax is present.
- Tuberculosis sequelae with negative ABF in sputum or bronchial aspirate specimens do not require treatment with antituberculosis drugs.
- Patients with inoperable non–small cell lung cancer less than 5 cm in size (T1-T2 N0M0) can be candidates for SBRT.
- SBRT for tumors greater than 5 cm in size is effective, but the risk of distant metastases remains.

Further Reading

1. Xu H, Koo HJ, Lee HN, et al. Lung cancer in patients with tuberculous fibrothorax and empyema: computed tomography and 18F-fluorodeoxyglucose positron emission tomography findings. *J Comput Assist Tomogr*. 2017;41(5):772–778.
2. Menon B, Nima G, Dogra V, Jha S. Evaluation of the radiological sequelae after treatment completion in new cases of pulmonary, pleural, and mediastinal tuberculosis. *Lung India*. 2015;32(3):241–245.
3. Meghji J, Simpson H, Squire SB, Mortimer K. A systematic review of the prevalence and pattern of imaging defined post-TB lung disease. *PLoS One*. 2016;11:e0161176.
4. Byrne AL, Marais BJ, Mitnick CD, Lecca L, Marks GB. Tuberculosis and chronic respiratory disease: a systematic review. *Int J Infect Dis*. 2015;32:138–146.
5. Kim HY, Song KS, Goo JM, et al. Thoracic sequelae and complications of tuberculosis. *Radiographics*. 2001;21(4):839–858.
6. Peterson J, Niles C, Patel A, et al. Stereotactic body radiotherapy for large (>5 cm) non-small-cell lung cancer. *Clin Lung Cancer*. 2017;18(4):396–400.
7. Nagata Y, Kimura T. Stereotactic body radiotherapy (SBRT) for stage I lung cancer. *Jpn J Clin Oncol*. 2018;48(5):405–409.
8. Febbo JA, Gaddikeri RS, Shah PN. Stereotactic body radiation therapy for early-stage non-small cell lung cancer: a primer for radiologists. *Radiographics*. 2018;38(5):1312–1336.

CHAPTER 5

Malignant Pleural Mesothelioma With Trapped Lung

Claudio Sorino ▪ Filippo Lococo ▪ Giampietro Marchetti ▪ Abdul Hamid Alraiyes

History of Present Illness

A 60-year-old man presented to the general practitioner for breathlessness and dry cough. The symptoms had arisen a few months earlier and had gradually worsened. Chest radiography revealed complete opacification of the right hemithorax, suggestive of massive pleural effusion (Fig. 5.1). Therefore he was urgently referred to an outpatient pulmonary clinic.

Past Medical History

The patient was a former smoker with a 15-pack-year history (about 10 cigarettes a day for 30 years) and had been exposed to asbestos 40 years earlier, when he started working as a brick-layer. He had never been hospitalized and did not take medications routinely.

Physical Examination and Early Clinical Findings

During pulmonary evaluation, the patient was alert and cooperative. He was afebrile and had mild hypoxemia (oxygen saturation [SpO$_2$] 92% on room air), tachycardia (heart rate 95 beats/min at rest), tachypnea (respiratory rate 25 breaths/min), and normal blood pressure (125/80 mm Hg). On chest examination, breath sounds were absent in all the right hemithorax, with dullness on percussion. No pallor, clubbing, and peripheral edema were observed. Chest ultrasonography confirmed the presence

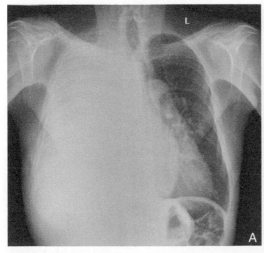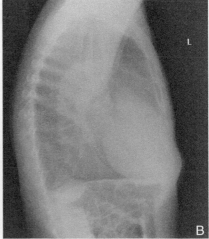

Fig. 5.1 Posteroanterior (A) and lateral (B) chest radiographs showing extensive right opacity, suggestive of massive pleural effusion with a slight mediastinal shift to the contralateral side.

41

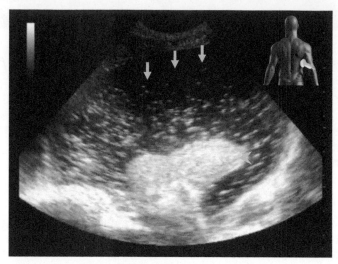

Fig. 5.2 Ultrasound appearance of the right hemothorax, demonstrating pleural effusion with multiple floating particles within the fluid (the so-called plankton sign, *arrows*), whereas the collapsed lung *(arrowhead)* showed only minimal movements.

of massive right pleural effusion, with floating particles inside the fluid and a poorly moving collapsed lung (Fig. 5.2). The patient was admitted to the pulmonology department for further workup.

Clinical Course

Blood test results were within normal limits. Hemoglobin was 14.6 g/dL, total leukocyte count was 8.660 cells/mm³, platelet count was 180.000 cells/μL, and international normalized ratio (INR) was 1.12. Electrocardiography (ECG) showed sinus rhythm.

Discussion Topic

Pulmonologist A

The pleural fluid is copious and probably thick. How about placing a large-bore chest tube?

Pulmonologist B

The pleural effusion is most likely caused by malignancy. I'm willing to perform thoracoscopy today so that we can explore the pleural cavity and perform pleural biopsies.

Pulmonologist A

Why not? Do you want computed tomography (CT) to be performed urgently?

Discussion Topic—cont'd

Pulmonologist B

Chest radiography and ultrasonography are enough for me. CT can be done after thoracoscopy.

Pulmonologist A

Will you attempt pleurodesis at the end of thoracoscopy?

Pulmonologist B

I usually wait for the frozen section of the pleural biopsy, which allows for a rapid microscopic analysis of the specimen. If this will confirm malignancy, I'll spray talc and then leave a chest tube with aspiration.

However, pleurodesis requires that the visceral and parietal pleurae be close. If the lung does not expand sufficiently, any pleurodesis attempt will be ineffective.

On the day of admission, medical thoracoscopy was performed. The patient received moderate sedation (intravenous 5 mg of midazolam and 50 μg of fentanyl) and local anesthesia (10 mL of 2% lidocaine), followed by analgesics (paracetamol 1000 mg three times daily and tramadol as needed).

Oxygen via nasal cannula was administered with 3 to 4 L/min to maintain SpO_2 values greater than 94%. A small incision (about 1 cm, parallel to the upper margin of the rib) was made in the fifth intercostal space along the midaxillary line. After penetration of the parietal pleura with a clamp, a trocar was introduced, and a rigid thoracoscope was placed through the trocar. A high amount of orange pleural fluid (2.8 L) was immediately drained. Visceral and parietal pleura were covered with easily desquamating yellow tissue. Many particles of similar tissue were floating in the pleural fluid as well (Fig. 5.3).

The lesions were extensively involving diaphragm, pulmonary apex, pericardium, and subclavian vessels.

Multiple biopsies were performed on the parietal pleura, and samples were sent for histopathological and microbiological examinations. At the end of the procedure, an attempt at talc poudrage was made, then a 24 French (Fr) chest tube was inserted through the same entry port and connected to a three-chamber unit. Suction (–20 cm H_2O) was applied for 3 days.

Chest radiography performed after thoracoscopy (Fig. 5.4) demonstrated right hydropneumothorax, with nonexpanded right lung. Chest computed tomography (CT) with contrast medium

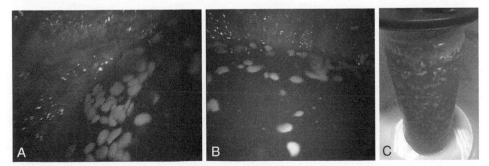

Fig. 5.3 Thoracoscopic view of pleura and pleural fluid demonstrating orange pleural fluid with floating yellow particles (A, B) and appearance of the pleural fluid in the suction canister (C).

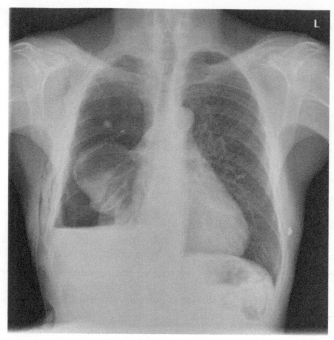

Fig. 5.4 Post-thoracoscopy posteroanterior chest radiograph, showing right hydropneumothorax with non-expanded lung.

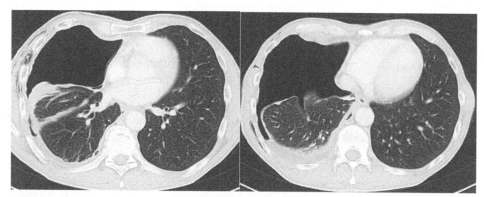

Fig. 5.5 Axial chest computed tomography (CT) scan (lung window setting) taken after thoracoscopy, showing right hydropneumothorax with air-fluid level, thickened pleural, and trapped lung.

(Fig. 5.5) confirmed the radiographic findings. Both the parietal and visceral pleurae were thickened at the costal, mediastinal, and diaphragmatic levels. Lymph node enlargement was present in the right tracheobronchial angle, right hilum, mediastinum, and subpleural fatty tissue. Some subcutaneous emphysema was present on the right side. Abdominal CT showed no metastatic lesions in the liver, spleen, pancreas, adrenals, kidneys, or bladder.

Histological examination of the pleural biopsy specimens revealed biphasic malignant mesothelioma (Fig. 5.6). The patient was discharged and subsequently re-evaluated as an outpatient after 2 weeks.

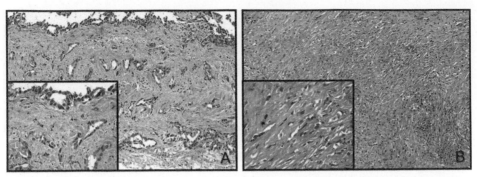

Fig. 5.6 Hematoxylin-eosin–stained sections (medium power) of pleural biopsies showing both epithelioid (A) and sarcomatoid (B) components. The epithelioid pattern typically has epithelioid cells with abundant eosinophilic cytoplasm, organized in tubular/pseudoacinar structures invading the surrounding collagenous stroma. The sarcomatous pattern is characterized by a hypercellular spindle cell neoplasm with elongated nuclei, numerous mitotic figures, and eosinophilic cytoplasm.

Discussion Topic

Pulmonologist A

Is the surgical treatment limited because of the extension of disease?

Thoracic surgeon

I regret to admit that it is so. The two main methods of surgery for pleural mesothelioma are the extrapleural pneumonectomy and pleurectomy with decortication. Both options should be dismissed because macroscopic complete resection is not possible.

Pulmonologist B

Do you think the patient can tolerate chemotherapy treatment?

Oncologist

The best way to answer this is by evaluating his performance status.

Follow-Up and Outcomes

Two weeks after discharge, the stitches at the drainage insertion site were removed. Despite some respiratory symptoms, the patient was able to carry on normal activity, but with some effort. His performance status was estimated to be 80% according to the Karnofsky Performance Score (KPS), corresponding to an Eastern Clinical Oncology Group PS (ECOG PS) score of 1.

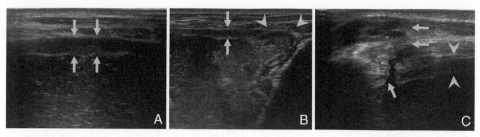

Fig. 5.7 Ultrasonography performed 12 months after diagnosis. (A) Thickening of the parietal pleura *(vertical arrows)* with persistent pleural effusion. (B) Involvement of the costophrenic recess *(arrowheads)* and thickening parietal pleura *(vertical arrows)*. (C) neoplastic infiltration of the thoracoscopy tract *(oblique and horizontal arrows)* and parietal pleura *(arrowheads)*.

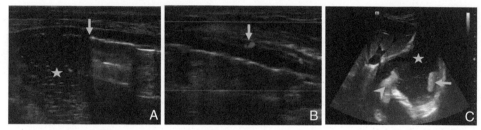

Fig. 5.8 Ultrasonography performed 18 months after diagnosis. (A) Air-fluid level *(vertical arrow)*, fluid with plankton sign *(star)*. (B) Evidence of vascularization (in color Doppler) in the infiltrated parietal pleura. (C) Local evolution with further pleural thickening *(horizontal arrow)*, collapsed lung *(arrowhead)*, and pleural effusion with plankton sign *(star)*.

First-line chemotherapy with a combination of cisplatin and pemetrexed was started. The disease showed stability in the first 6 months; however, at 12 months, the disease advanced locally, although with no distal metastasis. Chest ultrasonography performed at this stage of follow-up showed worsened thickening of the parietal pleura, involvement of the costophrenic recess, and clear infiltration of the thoracoscopy tract (Fig. 5.7). Subsequently, more pleural thickening and signs of tumor vascularization were observed (Fig. 5.8). With disease progression, the patient declined further chemotherapy. Two sessions of palliative thoracentesis were performed to relieve respiratory symptoms. The patient died 22 months after diagnosis.

Focus On

Medical Thoracoscopy

Medical thoracoscopy (MT), also known as *local anesthetic thoracoscopy* or *pleuroscopy,* is a minimally invasive endoscopic procedure performed under local anesthesia (infiltration of skin, subcutaneous tissue, intercostal muscle, and parietal pleura).

In contrast to video-assisted thoracoscopic surgery (VATS), patients typically receive moderate sedation and breathe spontaneously throughout the procedure, without positive pressure ventilation.

Focus On—cont'd

Through a single-port access, a trocar/introducer is inserted into the pleural cavity; then a rigid or semirigid thoracoscope is advanced. This allows for inspection of both the visceral and parietal pleural surfaces (directly or indirectly by video). By maneuvering the thoracoscope, the operator usually starts to examine the apex and then the costal pleura, the diaphragm, and the mediastinal pleura, ending back at the apex. Adequate assessment of the diaphragmatic pleura and costophrenic recesses is particularly important.

The thoracoscope has channels to aspirate and perform biopsies under direct visualization and to perform therapeutic procedures, such as talc poudrage and tunneled indwelling pleural catheter (TIPC) placement.

Consequently, MT has a particularly high diagnostic yield, comparable with that in VATS.

The semirigid thoracoscope has a distal tip that can be flexed and extended by 160 degrees and 130 degrees, respectively. It allows for easier maneuverability in the pleural space and a smaller incision. Moreover, most thoracic surgeons quickly learn how to use a semirigid thoracoscope because of its similarity to the flexible bronchoscope. However, rigid thoracoscopy provides larger biopsy samples and has a higher diagnostic yield. Safe thoracoscopy requires a large pleural cavity between the lung and the chest wall. In cases where there is little pleural fluid, a pneumothorax should be induced.

Focus On

Pleurodesis

Pleurodesis is a procedure that aims to obliterate the pleural space and prevent recurrent pleural effusion (mostly malignant) or pneumothorax.

The apposition of the visceral and parietal pleurae is necessary for successful pleurodesis. It can be achieved either by a physical method (e.g., mechanical abrasion, laser or argon beam coagulation during video-assisted thoracoscopic surgery [VATS]) or instillation of a chemical irritant into the pleural space (e.g., talc, bleomycin, tetracycline, iodopovidone), which induces inflammation and fibrosis.

Among the sclerosant agents for pleurodesis, talc is considered to have the best rate of success in malignant pleural effusions. It can be administered in slurry form (through the chest tube) or poudrage (through the thoracoscope).

Focus On

Assessment of Performance Status

General fitness, or performance status (PS), is often used as an indicator of a patient's ability to tolerate treatments, such as chemotherapy. Indeed, patients with a poor PS are associated with increased risk for chemotherapy toxicity and poor outcomes compared with patients with better PS.

The most common methods for assessing PS are the Karnofsky Performance Score (KPS) and the Eastern Clinical Oncology Group Performance Status (ECOG PS) scales.

The KPS scale ranges from 0 (dead) to 100 (normally active, without evidence of disease). The score assigned takes into consideration the patient's ability to perform daily activities and the level of assistance required.

The ECOG PS score has only six points, ranging from 0 (fully active) to 5 (dead). It is usually preferred by clinicians because it is simpler to use and has higher interobserver reproducibility.

Table 5.1 shows a commonly used method of comparison of the KPS and ECOG PS scores.

Many guidelines suggest that chemotherapy be avoided in patients with solid tumors who have an ECOG PS score of 3 or greater, corresponding to a KPS score of 40 or less.

For patients with an ECOG PS score of 2, lighter chemotherapy regimens are often suggested.

TABLE 5.1 ■ Comparison Between KPS and ECOG PS Scores

ECOG Performance Status	KPS Performance Status
0—Fully active, able to carry on all predisease performance without restriction	100—Normal, no complaints; no evidence of disease
	90—Able to carry on normal activity; minor signs or symptoms of disease
1—Restricted in physically strenuous activity but ambulatory and able to carry out work of a light or sedentary nature, e.g., light house work, office work	80—Normal activity with effort, some signs or symptoms of disease
	70—Cares for self but unable to carry on normal activity or to do active work
2—Ambulatory and capable of all self-care but unable to carry out any work activities; up and about more than 50% of waking hours	60—Requires occasional assistance but is able to care for most of personal needs
	50—Requires considerable assistance and frequent medical care
3—Capable of only limited self-care; confined to bed or chair more than 50% of waking hours	40—Disabled; requires special care and assistance
	30—Severely disabled; hospitalization is indicated although death not imminent
4—Completely disabled; cannot carry on any self-care; totally confined to bed or chair	20—Very ill; hospitalization and active supportive care necessary
	10—Moribund
5—Dead	0—Dead

ECOG PS, Eastern Cooperative Oncology Group, Performance Status; *KPS*, Karnofsky Performance Score.

LEARNING POINTS

- Malignant pleural mesothelioma (MPM) is a lethal disease with a poor prognosis.
- MPM is an aggressive cancer, with a propensity for seeding the tracts made by chest instrumentation.
- There is no evident role for prophylactic radiotherapy in MPM.
- Surgery should be reserved for select patients with a good performance status and for tumors of epithelioid/mixed histology if a specimen can be obtained from macroscopic complete resection.
- The combination of cisplatin and pemetrexed is the standard of care for inoperable MPM.

Further Reading

1. Alraiyes AH, Dhillon SS, Harris K, et al. Medical thoracoscopy: technique and application. *Pleura.* 2016;3:1–11.
2. Murthy V, Bessich JL. Medical thoracoscopy and its evolving role in the diagnosis and treatment of pleural disease. *J Thorac Dis.* 2017;9(Suppl 10):S1011–S1021.
3. Katzman D, Sterman DH. Updates in the diagnosis and treatment of malignant pleural mesothelioma. *Curr Opin Pulm Med.* 2018;24(4):319–326.
4. Bergamin S, Tio M, Stevens MJ. Prophylactic procedure tract radiotherapy for malignant pleural mesothelioma: a systematic review and meta-analysis. *Clin Transl Radiat Oncol.* 2018;13:38–43.
5. Mierzejewski M, Korczynski P, Krenke R, Janssen JP. Chemical pleurodesis—a review of mechanisms involved in pleural space obliteration. *Respir Res.* 2019;20(1):247.
6. Calati AM, Guglielmetti M, Sorino C, Caronno R. Video-assisted thoracic surgery as a diagnostic tool. In: *Diagnostic Evaluation of the Respiratory System.* New Delhi, India: Jaypee Brothers Medical Publishers; 2017;400–403.
7. Ricciardi S, Cardillo G, Zirafa CC, et al. Surgery for malignant pleural mesothelioma: an international guidelines review. *J Thorac Dis.* 2018;10(Suppl 2):S285–S292.

CHAPTER 6

Lung Adenocarcinoma With Diffuse Pleural Infiltration in a Young Nonsmoker Man

Hari Kishan Gonuguntla ■ Nitesh Gupta ■ Claudio Sorino ■ David Feller-Kopman

History of Present Illness

A 35-year-old Asian man was referred to the pulmonology department for shortness of breath and a dull pain in his right lateral chest. His symptoms, which had started 3 months earlier, were a nonproductive cough, mild chest discomfort on the right side, and gradually worsened dyspnea on exertion. Chest radiography (Fig. 6.1) revealed large pleural effusion on the right side without contralateral mediastinal shift; the effusion was nonloculated, as seen on chest ultrasonography (Fig. 6.2). The patient underwent thoracentesis, with about 1400 mL of dark straw-colored pleural fluid extracted. Biochemical analysis of the pleural fluid was consistent with exudate: lactate dehydrogenase (LDH) 353 units/L (serum LDH 189 units/L; ratio 1.86) and protein 3.8 g/L (serum protein 3 g/L; ratio 1.26). Cytological analysis showed lymphocyte predominance (71%), with no evidence of malignant cells. The pleural fluid level of adenosine deaminase (ADA) was 22.20 units/mL; and the smear microscopy and nucleic acid amplification test results for *Mycobacterium tuberculosis* (Xpert MTB/RIF) were negative. Ten days later, ultrasonography showed recurrence of pleural effusion.

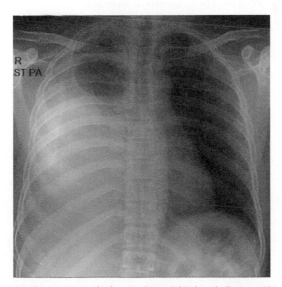

Fig. 6.1 Posteroanterior chest radiograph showing large right pleural effusion without mediastinal shift.

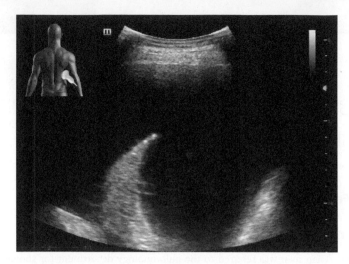

Fig. 6.2 Chest ultrasonography image showing right nonloculated pleural effusion.

Past Medical History

The patient was a goat farmer and a never-smoker. He had had no asbestos exposure, no known risk factors for tuberculosis, and no history of drug or alcohol abuse. The patient denied any recent weight loss or appetite reduction. He was not on any medication at the time of evaluation.

Discussion Topic

Pulmonologist A

The patient is a young man nonsmoker, with pleural fluid analysis of exudate. What could be the differential diagnosis?

Interventional pulmonologist

He had no fever or other signs of acute infection. However, tuberculosis (TB) should be considered because we are in an endemic region and because there was lymphocyte predominance in the pleural fluid.

Pulmonologist B

The low values of pleural adenosine deaminase (ADA) don't support TB, although the test is most helpful when ADA is greater than 45 units/mL. Other causes of exudative pleural effusion should also be considered.

Pulmonologist A

Could we place a chest tube and repeat the pleural fluid analysis for detection of malignant cells?

Discussion Topic—cont'd

Interventional pulmonologist

I think this may be a waste of time. The patient has already undergone the analysis with negative results. We should now perform targeted biopsies to obtain specimens for histological examination.

Pulmonologist B

Do you mean closed pleural biopsies or biopsies via thoracoscopy?

Interventional pulmonologist

The diagnostic yield of thoracoscopy is definitely higher than that of closed pleural biopsy, and the complication rate is lower as well. Hence I suggest we go ahead with thoracoscopy.

Physical Examination and Early Clinical Findings

The patient was referred directly to the interventional pulmonology department, with a request for medical thoracoscopy–guided biopsy. Upon admission, the patient was alert, cooperative, and afebrile. The room air oxygen saturation measured by pulse oximetry was 96%, heart rate was 70 beats/min, and blood pressure was 130/80 mm Hg. Physical examination revealed decreased movements of the right hemithorax, reduced tactile fremitus, stony-dull percussion in the right pulmonary field, and absent breath sounds. No lymphadenopathy, clubbing, or pallor was evident. Chest ultrasonography showed residual right pleural effusion. Routine blood tests showed hemoglobin (Hb) 15.20 g/dL, and total leukocyte count 7,040 cells/mm³, and normal differential count. Platelet count was 298,000 cells/μL, and the international normalized ratio (INR) was 1.16.

Computed tomography (CT) of the chest (Fig. 6.3) showed the presence of large right pleural effusion with mild pleural thickening. Lymph node enlargement was seen (levels 3, 4R, and 7), and no parenchymal abnormalities were evident.

Discussion Topic

Pulmonologist A

We should check that the patient has no contraindications for thoracoscopy.

Interventional pulmonologist

The only major contraindication for thoracoscopy is lack of pleural space resulting from extensive adhesions of the pleural layer. Here the lung is far away from the chest wall.

Continued

Discussion Topic—cont'd

Pulmonologist A

Perfect. Are there other factors that make it necessary to postpone the procedure?

Pulmonologist B

No. The patient is young, medically stable, has only slight hypoxemia and no hypercapnia. He has no heart disease. He does not routinely take drugs, specifically anticoagulants or antiplatelet agents. Kidney function is normal, and the platelet count and international normalized ratio (INR) results are within normal limits.

Pulmonologist A

Is the procedure completely painless?

Pulmonologist B

The patient will undergo sedation to reduce discomfort. He may experience a small amount of pain during local anesthesia, mainly when the needle penetrates the skin and the parietal pleura.

Interventional pulmonologist

He could feel brief discomfort or pain when biopsy of the parietal pleura is performed or when talc is insufflated. This can be avoided if we give additional sedative or analgesics, such as intrapleural lidocaine spray, before the procedure.

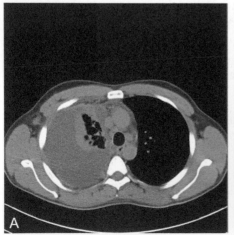 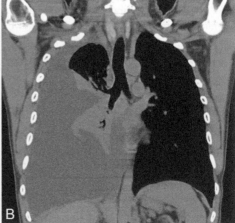

Fig. 6.3 Axial (A) and coronal (B) chest computed tomography (CT) scans showing the presence of large right pleural effusion and mild pleural thickening.

Clinical Course

The patient underwent rigid thoracoscopy under moderate sedation (intravenous midazolam and fentanyl). Thoracoscopic examination revealed a diffuse white, nodular, flat growth on the parietal pleura at the costodiaphragmatic level and flat tumor infiltrations on the visceral pleura among the upper lobe, middle lobe, and lower lobe (Fig. 6.4). Multiple biopsy specimens were obtained from the parietal pleura for histopathological and microbiological examinations. Subsequently, chemical pleurodesis was performed with talc poudrage. A total of 4 g of talc was atomized and insufflated into the pleural space through a catheter placed in the working channel of the thoracoscope. Uniform distribution of the talc on all pleural surfaces was confirmed by direct visualization. At the conclusion of the procedure, a chest tube was inserted to drain residual air and fluid from the pleural cavity. Five days after the procedure, no air leakage was evident, and drained fluid was less than 100 mL per day; therefore the chest tube was removed and the patient discharged.

Histological examination of pleural biopsy specimens (Fig. 6.5) showed irregular glandular structures infiltrating the stroma. The cells show nuclear atypia and cytoplasmic vacuoles. On immunohistochemistry, the tumor cells were positive for thyroid transcription factor 1 (TTF-1) and negative for p-40. These features suggested metastases of lung adenocarcinoma. The subsequent molecular analysis was positive for the anaplastic lymphoma kinase gene *ALK (D5F3)*

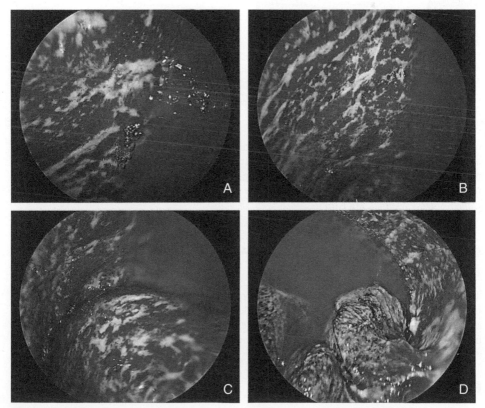

Fig. 6.4 Pleuroscopic view of parietal pleura, showing white nodular and flat tumor growth on the anterior chest wall pleura (A to D).

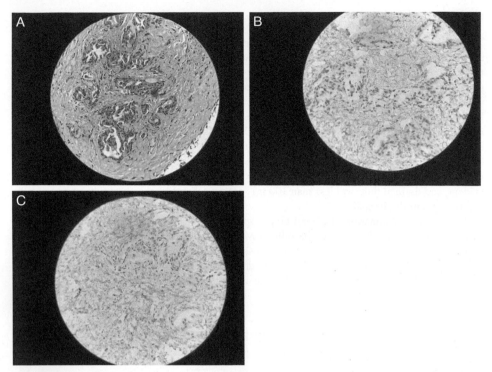

Fig. 6.5 Microscopic appearance of metastatic lung adenocarcinoma on pleural biopsies. (A) Hematoxylin-eosin–stained section. (B) Positive staining for thyroid transcription factor 1 (TTF-1) on immunohistochemistry. (C) Negative staining for calretinin (mesothelial marker) on immunohistochemistry.

mutation. The patient was evaluated for distant metastasis through brain CT, abdominal CT, and bone scanning, all of which yielded negative results. Because of pleural involvement, however, the patient's disease was staged as non–small-cell lung carcinoma (NSCLC) stage IV, according to the tumor–node–metastasis (TNM) classification per the *American Joint Committee on Cancer (AJCC) Cancer Staging Manual,* 8th edition.

Recommended Therapy and Further Indications at Discharge

The postoperative course was uneventful, and the patient was started on crizotinib, a kinase inhibitor, in tablet form, 250 mg two times a day, as indicated for metastasized ALK-positive or reactive oxygen species 1 (ROS1)–positive NSCLC. The oncologist planned continuation of the drug until unsatisfactory response or disease progression on chemotherapy.

Follow-Up and Outcomes

Three weeks after discharge, the patient underwent follow-up chest radiography (Fig. 6.6), which demonstrated no evidence of pleural effusion, suggesting successful pleurodesis.

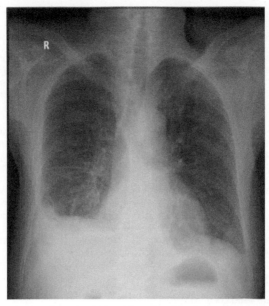

Fig. 6.6 Posteroanterior chest radiograph obtained 3 weeks after discharge showing good expansion of the right lung.

Focus On

Rigid and Semirigid Thoracoscopy

Thoracoscopy employs an optical system to examine the pleural cavity and perform diagnostic and therapeutic procedures. It should be considered in patients with pleural effusion that remain undiagnosed despite pleural fluid analysis and/or closed pleural biopsy (approximately 25% of exudative pleural effusions).

Thoracoscopy has traditionally been divided into surgical thoracoscopy (video-assisted thoracoscopic surgery [VATS]) and medical thoracoscopy (also known as *pleuroscopy*). VATS is typically performed by thoracic surgeons, with the patients under general anesthesia and single-lung ventilation. Medical thoracoscopy is usually performed by pulmonologists, with the patients under moderate sedation and local anesthesia.

The instruments available for medical thoracoscopy include rigid or semirigid (or flexi-rigid) thoracoscopes. A rigid thoracoscopy is made of a stainless steel rigid telescope of about 30 cm in length and a diameter of 4 to 12 mm. The semirigid pleuroscope has a proximal rigid shaft (about 20 cm) and a flexible distal tip (about 5 cm) that allows up and down angulations. The handle of the semirigid pleuroscope is similar to that of a flexible bronchoscope. Both rigid and semirigid thoracoscopes are placed into the pleural space through a trocar.

The crucial distinction is the ability to navigate and reach various parts of the pleural cavity. The rigid thoracoscope provides better vision, aiding anatomical identification inside the pleural cavity, providing large-size biopsy samples using a single port of entry, and also assisting biopsies of hard/firm lesions. The semirigid thoracoscopy, with the "look and feel of a bronchoscope," provides lateral vision conveniently or even retro visualization of the point of entry.

Rigid thoracoscopy has similar diagnostic yield compared with semirigid thoracoscopy in exudative pleural effusions. However, larger biopsy samples can be obtained during rigid thoracoscopy. In the current era of molecular therapy for lung cancer, the larger biopsy specimen may offer an added advantage in the assessment of pleural tumor burden.

Medical thoracoscopy, either by rigid or semirigid instruments, is a safe procedure in experienced hands. The overall mortality rate is less than 0.5%. The major complications are quite rare and include empyema, severe bleeding, port site metastasis, persistent air leak, and pneumonia. Minor complications include pyrexia, subcutaneous emphysema, skin infection, and minor hemorrhage. In terms of periprocedure pain, larger trocars can cause more significant discomfort and new smaller rigid thoracoscopes allow smaller incisions. The decision to use either of the instruments is primarily determined based on equipment availability.

Focus On

Macroscopic Pleural Aspect of Malignancy at Thoracoscopy

The inspection of the pleural cavity through a thoracoscope should be first performed from a distance able to allow a panoramic view and then from a distance of 1 to 2 cm from the surfaces. In the case of a large pleural effusion, the fluid should be aspirated completely (air should be allowed to enter the pleural space through the cannula to replace the aspirated volume, thus maintaining normal intrapleural pressure and prevent re-expansion edema). Fibrinous strands interfering with a clear view should be removed.

Macroscopic examination allows for recognition of the pattern of pleural involvement and also helps in the identification of a target site for biopsy. In its normal state, the parietal pleura is thin and transparent, allowing visualization of underlying diaphragm, ribs, fat, and vessels.

Several malignancies occur with pleural masses, nodules, plaques, adhesions. Extensive pleural disease is easy to recognize, but localized disease or small, isolated lesions may go unnoticed. Diffuse thickening of the pleura, similar to a rind, encases the lung and is one of the most common appearances of malignant pleural mesothelioma (MPM). MPM can also form nodules in the parietal pleura, mainly over the diaphragmatic surfaces, and invade hyalinized pleural plaques. Only rarely does MPM occur as a single mass without diffuse thickening or satellite nodules.

Localized pleural anomalies include granulomas, which usually are 1 to 3 mm in diameter and can be caused by sarcoidosis or tuberculosis. Pleural nodules may have different sizes and shapes. The finding of variably sized nodules is highly suggestive of malignancy, whereas uniformly sized nodules should increase suspicion of tuberculosis. The nodules can be grape-like, cauliflower-like lesions, fused into masses or diffused. A subtle reticular pattern may be suggestive of lymphangitis.

The lung appears like a cone, narrowing at the apex. The visceral pleural surface is transparent. When the lung is healthy, the surface is pink and soft, with a reticular pattern demarcating the pulmonary lobules. Black anthracotic pigments scattered over the surface are often observed in patients exposed to carbon-containing dust particles. Areas of atelectasis are purplish-red with a definite edge. The identification of nodules protruding from the lung surface is highly suggestive of malignancy.

LEARNING POINTS

- When recurrent unilateral pleural effusion occurs, malignancy is a possible diagnosis even in young adult nonsmokers and in tuberculosis-endemic regions.
- Rigid thoracoscopy allows for obtaining large biopsy specimens that aid in the assessment of pleural tumor burden and for molecular analysis.
- Macroscopic examination of the pleura must be performed meticulously, especially in localized diseases.
- Pleural manometry may help estimate the ability of the lung to expand during therapeutic thoracentesis and predict pleurodesis success.
- Talc is the best agent for chemical pleurodesis, and poudrage and slurry are equally effective.

Further Reading

1. DeBiasi EM, Feller-Kopman D. Physiologic basis of symptoms in pleural disease. *Semin Respir Crit Care Med.* 2019;40(3):305–313.
2. Hooper C, Lee YC, Maskell NBTS Pleural Guideline Group. Investigation of a unilateral pleural effusion in adults: British Thoracic Society Pleural Disease Guideline 2010. *Thorax.* 2010;65(Suppl 2):ii4–ii17.
3. Loddenkemper R, Mathur PN, Noppen M, et al. *Medical Thoracoscopy/Pleuroscopy. Manual and Atlas.* Stuttgart and New York: Thieme; 2011.
4. Bibby AC, Dorn P, Psallidas I, et al. ERS/EACTS statement on the management of malignant pleural effusions. *Eur Respir J.* 2018;52:1800349.

5. Dhooria S, Singh N, Agarwal AN, Gupta D, Agarwal R. A randomized trial comparing the diagnostic yield of rigid and semirigid thoracoscopy in undiagnosed pleural effusion. *Respir Care.* 2014;59(5):756–764.

6. Rozman A, Camlek L, Marc-Malovrh M, Triller N, Kern I. Rigid versus semi-rigid thoracoscopy for diagnosis of pleural disease: a randomized pilot study. *Respirology.* 2013;18(4):704–710.

7. Grabczak EM, Krenke R, Zielinska-Krawczyk M, Light RW. Pleural manometry in patients with pleural diseases—the usefulness in clinical practice. *Respir Med.* 2018;145:230–236.

8. Bhatnagar R, Laskawiec-Szkonter M, Piotrowska HEG, et al. Evaluating the efficacy of thoracoscopy and talc poudrage versus pleurodesis using talc slurry (TAPPS trial): protocol of an open-label randomised controlled trial. *BMJ Open.* 2014;4:e007045.

9. Wahidi MM, Reddy C, Yarmus L, et al. Randomized trial of pleural fluid drainage frequency in patients with malignant pleural effusions. The ASAP trial. *Am J Respir Crit Care Med.* 2017;195:1050–1057.

10. Hu K, Chopra A, Huggins JT, Nanchal R. Pleural manometry: techniques, applications, and pitfalls. *J Thorac Dis.* 2020;20(5):2759–2770.

11. Chopra A, Judson MA, Doelken P, et al. The relationship of pleural manometry with postthoracentesis chest radiographic findings in malignant pleural effusion. *Chest.* 2020;157(2):421–426.

12. Dresler CM, Olak J, Herndon JE, 2nd, et al. Phase III intergroup study of talc poudrage vs talc slurry sclerosis for malignant pleural effusion. *Chest.* 2005;127(3):909–915.

13. Bhatnagar R, Maskell NA. Delivery of talc for pleurodesis of malignant pleural effusions—reply. *JAMA.* 2020;323(18):1855–1856.

CHAPTER 7

Chylothorax Associated With Indolent Follicular Lymphoma

Filippo Lococo ▪ Claudio Sorino ▪ Giampietro Marchetti
▪ David Feller-Kopman

History of Present Illness

A 62-year-old Caucasian woman experienced subacute onset of dyspnea. Chest radiography showed the presence of massive right pleural effusion (Fig. 7.1). Therefore she was referred to the pulmonology department.

Past Medical History

The patient had a history of indolent follicular lymphoma with multiple thoracic and abdominal lesions. She had no history of smoking or alcohol abuse, and her previous medical history was otherwise unremarkable.

The patient underwent radiotherapy and first-line chemoimmunotherapy with the rituximab, cyclophosphamide, hydroxydaunomycin (doxorubicin), Oncovin (vincristine), and prednisone (R-CHOP) regimen for 4 weeks. Subsequent [18]F- fluorodeoxyglucose (FDG) positron emission tomography/computed tomography (PET/CT), performed for restaging purposes, showed the

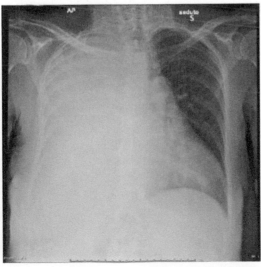

Fig. 7.1 Chest radiograph showing massive right-sided pleural effusion with contralateral trachea and mediastinum deviation.

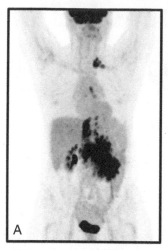
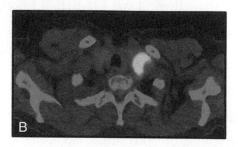

Fig. 7.2 (A) Frontal positron emission tomography (PET) scan showing intense fluorodeoxyglucose (FDG) uptake in multiple localizations of lymphoma at the level of abdominal lymph nodes and in the left supraclavicular fossa. (B) Combined PET and computed tomography (CT) axial image showing a detail of the supraclavicular lesion.

persistence of intense uptake (maximum standard uptake value [SUV_{max}] 10.7) at the level of the left supraclavicular fossa and in several abdominal lymph nodes (Fig. 7.2, A and B). Consequently the treatment was continued. There was no evidence of pleural effusion at that time (1 month before the current presentation).

Physical Examination and Early Clinical Findings

At the time of admission, the patient was afebrile, oxygen saturation (SpO_2), measured with pulse oximetry, was 95% on room air, heart rate was 92 beats/minute, and blood pressure 120/70 mm Hg.

Physical examination revealed a marked reduction in breath sounds and the presence of tactile fremitus and dullness to percussion in almost all of the right pulmonary field.

Chest ultrasonography showed anechoic right pleural effusion without any significant septation (Fig. 7.3). Routine blood tests showed moderate leukocytosis (white blood cell [WBC] count

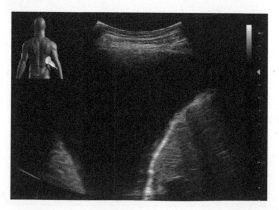

Fig. 7.3 Right chest ultrasonography scan showing a large anechoic supradiaphragmatic area caused by free-flowing pleural effusion.

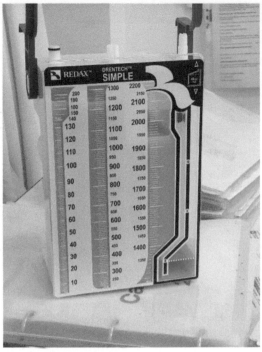

Fig. 7.4 Turbid appearance of the pleural effusion drained by a small-bore chest tube. Used with the permission of REDAX.

14,550/mm³) and a normal differential count. Electrolyte concentration and the results of the liver and kidney function tests were normal.

Clinical Course

An ultrasound-guided small-bore chest drain (12-French [Fr]) was placed, and about 1900 mL of cloudy pleural, nonmalodorous fluid was evacuated (Fig. 7.4). The procedure was well tolerated, and the pleural fluid was sent to the laboratory for analysis.

Discussion Topic

Wow, see what the pleural fluid looks like!

Pulmonologist A

It is cloudy and creamy. Given the patient's medical history, it could be chylothorax!

Pulmonologist B

Continued

Discussion Topic—cont'd

Pulmonologist A

Chylothorax should be milky, right?

Pulmonologist B

It can be milky but also serous or serosanguinous. The absence of milky appearance does not exclude chylothorax!

Pulmonologist A

Empyema should be excluded.

Pulmonologist B

I agree! When I smelled the fluid, however, it didn't smell like pus. We will send fluid samples for physicochemical examination, cytology, and culture. We will also ask for additional tests, such as white blood cell count differential, total triglycerides, and cholesterol levels.

Chemical analysis of the pleural fluid revealed the following: pH 7.42, glucose 43 mg/dL, triglyceride 728 mg/dL, and cholesterol 70 mg/dL. Pleural fluid WBC count showed 78% of lymphocytes.

These findings confirmed the diagnosis of chylothorax. Conservative treatment, consisting of total parenteral nutrition and subcutaneous administration of octreotide (at a dose of 100 μg every 8 hours for 3 days and subsequently titrated up to 200 μg every 8 hours, over a 6-day period), was started. Chest CT showed small residual right-sided pleural effusion but no lung parenchymal involvement (Fig. 7.5). In the subsequent 10 days, the amount of drained fluid remarkably decreased (from 1.2 L/day to 0.8 L/day), although it persisted. The macroscopic and physicochemical characteristics were consistent with the persistence of chylothorax.

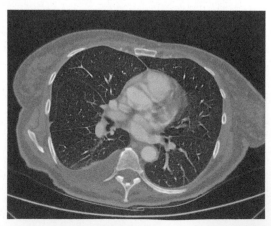

Fig. 7.5 Chest computed tomography (CT) scan showing residual right pleural effusion without other intrathoracic abnormalities.

Discussion Topic

Pulmonologist A

We found chylothorax in a woman with lymphoma. Could you help us?

Thoracic surgeon

Certainly. She is already fasting, right?

Pulmonologist A

Yes, but she still produces about 1 L of chyle every day.

Thoracic surgeon

So I think we'll try a surgical approach.

A surgical approach, with the aim of interrupting the chyle leak into the chest cavity, was indicated. About 1 hour before surgery, an oral cream was administered to increase chyle flow and to enhance visualization of the leak. The patient then underwent video-assisted thoracoscopic surgery (VATS) under general anesthesia. At surgery, the posterior mediastinal pleura was visualized, and a moderate but diffuse leak of chyle was observed at this site (Fig. 7.6).

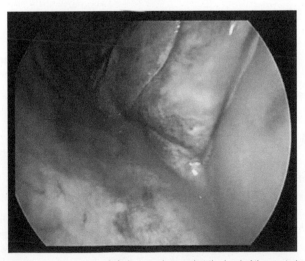

Fig. 7.6 Thoracoscopic view: a diffuse leak of chyle was observed at the level of the posterior mediastinal pleura.

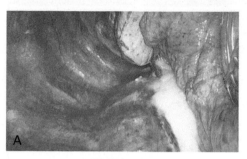
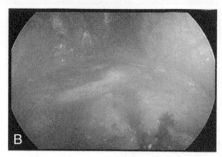

Fig. 7.7 Thoracoscopic view. (A) Glue placement. (B) Talc poudrage.

Because a diffuse chyle leakage was observed, the thoracic surgeon decided to not perform thoracic duct ligation but opted to spray a fibrin sealant (human fibrinogen/human thrombin, EVICEL, 5 mL) at the point of the greatest spill, followed by talc poudrage (4 g) (Fig. 7.7, A and B) with the final aim of achieving complete pleurodesis and to reduce the risk of recurrence of chylothorax.

Discharge, Follow-Up, and Outcomes

Total parenteral nutrition and octreotide therapy were continued postoperatively for 4 days; the chemical laboratory test on the pleural fluid demonstrated absence of chyle in the pleural fluid on postoperative days 2 and 6 after resumption of a normal diet. No pleural fluid was present 4 weeks after surgery; chemotherapy was resumed, and complete remission of lymphoma was achieved 3 months later.

Discussion Topic

Pulmonologist A

Could preoperative lymphatic scintigraphy be useful before thoracoscopy to visualize the area of chyle leak?

Thoracic surgeon

Data concerning the accuracy of this imaging tool are scarce and conflicting. Moreover, it was not available at our center. So we adopted another approach.

Pulmonologist A

Oral administration of cream?

Thoracic surgeon

Exactly! Administrated until 6 hours before the procedure, it increases chyle flow during surgical exploration. This can also be done intraoperatively via a nasogastric tube. In this case, the leak was not localized in a single area.

Discussion Topic—cont'd

Pulmonologist A

This increases the risk of recurrence?

Thoracic surgeon

Probably yes. So we decided to place glue to achieve better closure of the mediastinal pleura. The procedure was then completed with chemical pleurodesis to minimize the risk of recurrence of pleural effusion.

Focus On

Chest Tube Types and Sizes

Many types of chest tubes exist: straight, angled, and coiled at the end ("pig-tail"). They can be made of different materials and have several holes along the side and the tip and a radiopaque stripe with a gap that serves to mark the most proximal drain hole ("sentinel" hole). Some tubes have a double lumen, the small one usually being used for irrigation.

Chest tubes are usually classified according to their size. The French system is the most used worldwide. The size is expressed in *Ch* (Charrière, from the name of the creator) or more simply in *Fr* (French, from the country where Charrière lived). The Ch or the Fr number corresponds to the circumference of the catheter. This can be estimated in millimeters by dividing the "French number" by Pi (approximately 3). Therefore a 24-Fr tube has an outer diameter of approximately 8 mm.

Focus On

Chylothorax: Etiology and Diagnosis

Chylothorax is the accumulation of chyle (lymphatic fluid of intestinal origin) in the pleural space. It is caused by damage or obstruction of the thoracic duct or its tributaries.

The etiology of chylothorax can be traumatic or nontraumatic. Thoracic surgical procedures (esophagectomy, pulmonary resection with lymph node dissection, surgery for congenital heart disease) account for the majority of cases of traumatic chylothorax.

Among nontraumatic chylothoraces, malignancies (mainly lymphoma, chronic lymphocytic leukemia, and metastatic cancer) are the leading causes.

The pathophysiology of chylothorax associated with lymphoma is still unclear. In few cases, direct infiltration of the thoracic duct by cancer has been postulated, but more frequently, this condition is related to increased pressure in the thoracic duct causing retrograde flow of chyle via the microleaks of the thoracic duct or via the lymphatics of the parietal pleura into the pleural cavity.

Because the thoracic duct curves left at the level of the fifth or sixth thoracic vertebra (Fig. 7.8), an injury to the duct below this level usually produces right chylothorax, whereas one above this level produces left chylothorax.

The final diagnosis of chylothorax in patients with immunological defects or a history of neoplasm can be challenging. Chylothorax is typically milky or opalescent. It must be distinguished from cholesterol effusions, which have a similar appearance but different etiologies and therapies. Some chylothoraces can be serosanguinous, so a differential diagnosis that includes pleural empyema is necessary as well. The definitive diagnosis is substantially based on lab chemical results.

Pleural fluid triglyceride concentration greater than 110 mg/dL confirms the diagnosis of chylothorax. However, a value less than 50 mg/dL provides strong support that the patient does not have chylothorax. Lipoprotein electrophoresis can assist in diagnosis, especially in patients with pleural fluid triglyceride levels between 110 mg/dL and 50 mg/dL, because the presence of chylomicrons in the pleural fluid confirms chylothorax. Moreover, chylothoraces usually have low cholesterol levels (< 200 mg/dL or 5.18 mmol/L) and alkaline pH (7.40–7.80), whereas cholesterol effusions have elevated pleural fluid cholesterol levels and low triglyceride levels.

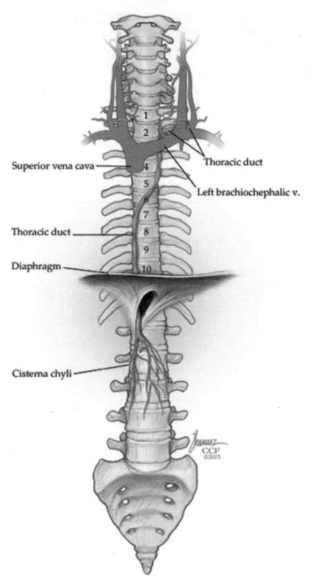

Fig. 7.8 Course of the thoracic duct from the cisternae chyli, up the right chest, crossing to the left side at around the fifth-sixth thoracic vertebra. (From Derakhshan A, Lubelski D, Steinmetz MP, et al. Thoracic duct injury following cervical spine surgery: a multicenter retrospective review. *Global Spine J*. 2017; 7[1 Suppl]:115S-119S.). Reprinted with permission, Cleveland Clinic Center for Medical Art & Photography © 2003-2020. All Rights Reserved.

Focus On

Treatment of Chylothorax

The optimal treatment for chylothorax is being strongly debated and still not defined clearly in the literature. A conservative approach often starts with a low-fat diet or a high–medium chain triglyceride–diet. If this is not effective, total parenteral nutrition and subcutaneous administration of octreotide can be tried. The duration of this approach could be protracted for weeks but only if the amount of chyle leak is not greater than approximately 1000 mL/day. With large (usually defined as > 1000 mL/day) or even moderate (500–800 mL/day) output of chylothorax that is protracted for several days, a surgical approach is often recommended. Various procedures have been proposed. Ligation of the thoracic duct at the level of the thoracic tract is usually recommended first, especially when direct visualization of the anatomical defect is possible during surgery. In other cases, when the chyle leak is diffuse to the entire posterior mediastinal region with no clear visualization of a leak, another approach (i.e., pleurodesis) could be used despite controversial results in the literature. Lymphangiography with thoracic duct embolization can be attempted, although many centers do not have experience with this specialized technique.

LEARNING POINTS

- When cloudy pleural effusion is found, chylothorax should be considered in the differential diagnosis, along with pleural empyema and cholesterol effusion.
- The final diagnosis of chylothorax is usually confirmed by the presence of high pleural fluid triglyceride concentration.
- Conservative treatment is usually effective in chylothorax production less than 500 to 800 mL/day.
- A surgical approach (generally after a fat-free diet) is often required for chylothorax production greater than 800 to 1000 mL/day.
- The ligation of the thoracic duct is the main surgical procedure in chylothorax, but another approach (i.e., pleurodesis) can be proposed when the chyle leak is diffuse.

Further Reading

1. Ismail NA, Gordon J, Dunning J. The use of octreotide in the treatment of chylothorax following cardiothoracic surgery. *Interact Cardiovasc Thorac Surg*. 2015;20(6):848–854.
2. Janjetovic S, Janning M, Daukeva L, Bokemeyer C, Fiedler W. Chylothorax in a patient with Hodgkin's lymphoma: a case report and review of the literature. *Tumori*. 2013;99(3):e96–e99.
3. Simmgen M, Newlands ES, Southcott BM, Vigushin DM. Bilateral chylothorax due to retrosternal goiter in a patient with non-Hodgkin's lymphoma. *Med Oncol*. 2001;18(2):153–157.
4. Bender B, Murthy V, Chamberlain RS. The changing management of chylothorax in the modern era. *Eur J Cardiothorac Surg*. 2016;49(1):18–24.
5. Mares DC, Mathur PN. Medical thoracoscopic talc pleurodesis for chylothorax due to lymphoma: a case series. *Chest*. 1998;114(3):731–735.
6. Vida VL, Padalino MA, Barzon E, Stellin G. Efficacy of fibrinogen/thrombin-coated equine collagen patch in controlling lymphatic leaks. *J Card Surg*. 2012;27(4):441–442.
7. Venuta F, Diso D, Anile M, Rendina EA, Onorati I. Chest tubes: generalities. *Thorac Surg Clin*. 2017;27(1):1–5.
8. Mahmood K, Wahidi MM. Straightening out chest tubes: what size, what type, and when. *Clin Chest Med*. 2013;34(1):63–71.
9. Cooke DT, David EA. Large-bore and small-bore chest tubes: types, function, and placement. *Thorac Surg Clin*. 2013;23(1):17–24.

PART II

Infections

CHAPTER 8

Relapsing Unilateral Pleural Effusion Due to Unrecognized Tuberculosis

Claudio Sorino ■ David Feller-Kopman ■ Giampietro Marchetti ■ Michele Mondoni

History of Present Illness

A 35-year-old Caucasian woman went to the emergency room for right chest pain, tachycardia, and low-grade fever (37.5° C [99.5° F]). The symptoms had begun a couple of weeks earlier and had gotten progressively worse.

Past Medical History

The patient worked as a general practitioner, never smoked, and had a history of mammary fibro-adenomas and polycystic ovary syndrome. Six years earlier, she had undergone cholecystectomy for gallstones. She had one previous pregnancy with delivery by cesarean birth 2 years earlier, and she breastfed her baby for 15 months.

She probably had a limited amount of exposure to asbestos (it was present in the roof of the home where she had lived in the first 20 years of her life).

Physical Examination and Early Clinical Findings

A reduction in breath sounds and dullness to percussion were found at the right lower part of the chest. Arterial blood gas (ABG) analysis in room air showed hypoxemia and hypocapnia: pH 7.45; partial pressure of oxygen (PaO$_2$) 65 mm Hg; and partial pressure of carbon dioxide (PaCO$_2$) 29 mm Hg. Chest radiography revealed unilateral right-sided pleural effusion, without pulmonary parenchymal lesions; no left pleural effusion; and no pathological mediastinal findings (Fig. 8.1).

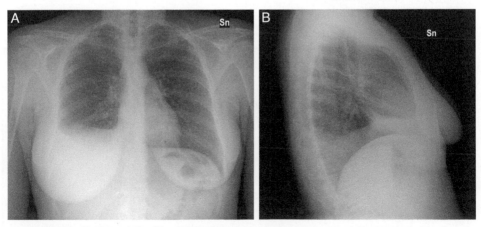

Fig. 8.1 Posteroanterior (A) and lateral (B) chest radiographs showing right pleural effusion.

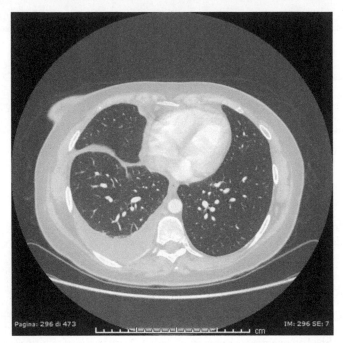

Fig. 8.2 Axial chest computed tomography (CT) scan (lung window level) showing right pleural effusion extending into the major fissure.

Blood tests showed a slight increase in the inflammation indices (C-reactive protein [CRP]: 32 mg/L; normal values < 5 mg/L), absence of leukocytosis (white blood cell [WBC] count: 8,030 cells/μL).

Well's criteria for pulmonary embolism were applied, and the patient was determined to be at low risk. Because D-dimer was not negative (644 ng/mL; normal values < 500 ng/mL), the patient underwent computed tomography pulmonary angiography (CTPA), which did not show pulmonary thromboembolism and confirmed right pleural effusion with a maximum thickness of approximately 35 mm (Fig. 8.2). Three very small nodules (maximum diameter approximately 3 mm) along the major fissure were identified. The patient was admitted to the internal medicine unit.

Discussion Topic

Infection is the most probable cause of the patient's symptoms. I would start empirical antibiotic therapy.

Internist

Pleural involvement without significant lung injury is not common. Thoracentesis would help clarify the diagnosis.

Pulmonologist

Discussion Topic—cont'd

Internist

We could wait a few days and see the response to therapy, reserving thoracentesis if the pleural effusion persists. Because the patient is suffering from chest pain, I would also give analgesics and glucocorticoids.

Pulmonologist

The attempt to obtain an etiological diagnosis should be made. Moreover, we should also perform investigations for noninfectious causes. Does the patient have sputum?

Internist

No, she doesn't. We can perform serology and urinary antigen detection tests.

Pulmonologist

Tuberculin skin test for detecting latent *Mycobacterium tuberculosis* infection is also necessary.

Clinical Course

Empirical therapy, including broad-spectrum antibiotics (piperacillin/tazobactam 4 g/0,5 g intravenously every 8 hours, plus oral levofloxacin 500 mg per day), systemic glucocorticoids (methylprednisolone 20 mg intravenously every 8 hours), and analgesics (paracetamol as needed), was begun.

Bedside thoracic ultrasonography showed only small right pleural effusion, which further reduced in the subsequent days. Therefore thoracentesis was not performed. Further blood tests showed positivity for anti-*Mycoplasma pneumoniae* immunoglobulin M (IgM). Results of screening tests for autoimmune disorders were negative (absence of antinuclear antigens [ANA], extractable nuclear antigens [ENA], proteinase 3 [PR3] and myeloperoxidase [MPO] anti-neutrophil cytoplasm antibodies [ANCA]).

Some tumor markers were assayed (carcinoembryonic antigen [CEA], cancer antigen [CA] 125, CA 15-3, CA 19-9, cytokeratin fragment [CYFRA] 21.1, neuron-specific enolase [NSE]), with an increase only in CA 125 (121 units/mL; normal values < 35). However, this marker is nonspecific and frequently increased in patients with pleural effusion.

A tuberculin skin test with five tuberculin units produced a reaction of 5 mm of induration after 72 hours. This is usually considered negative in people without known risk factors for tuberculosis (TB). However, QuantiFERON TB GOLD was prudently executed, but the result was not immediately available.

The patient experienced slow but progressive clinical improvement, with normalization of the inflammatory indices, resolution of the hypoxemia, and reduction in the amount of pleural effusion, as demonstrated by chest radiography and ultrasonography.

Recommended Therapy and Further Indications at Discharge

The patient was discharged after 10 days of hospitalization with the diagnosis of right pleuro-pneumonia caused by *Mycoplasma pneumoniae*.

The following home therapy was prescribed:

Levofloxacin 500 mg per day until reaching a total of 14 days of therapy.

Methylprednisolone 16 mg per day, with tapering every 3 days and discontinuation in 9 days

Outpatient follow-up after hospital discharge was suggested, with a control chest radiography after 4 weeks.

Follow-Up and Outcomes

Some days before the scheduled control, the patient went again to the emergency room because of high fever with shivering and chest pain. Chest radiography showed recurrence of right pleural effusion. Blood tests showed a WBC count 13,200 cells/µL (neutrophils 88%) and CRP 262.1 mg/L. The previously performed QuantiFERON TB test result was positive. The patient was admitted to the infectious disease unit.

Discussion Topic

Infectious disease specialist

A positive result from the QuantiFERON TB test allows for diagnosis of latent tuberculosis.

Attempts to identify an active disease should be made.

Pulmonologist

Identifying the presence of mycobacteria or their genetic material in biological samples is essential to evaluate the presence of active tuberculosis.

Infectious disease specialist

Organism isolation is important not only for definitive diagnosis but also for determining drug susceptibility.

Several investigations were performed to obtain biological samples for microscopy, cultures, and nucleic acid–based amplification test (NAAT).

First, a gastric aspirate sample was analyzed. Fasting, early morning specimens (5–10 mL on 3 consecutive days) were collected to obtain sputum swallowed during sleep. Both microscopy and research of ribosomal ribonucleic acid (r-RNA) of *Mycobacterium tuberculosis* complex (MTC) by

NAAT (polymerase chain reaction [PCR]) on gastric aspirate yielded negative results. Given the long waiting times for culture results (often up to 30–40 days), the patient underwent bronchoscopy with bronchoalveolar lavage. No macroscopic alteration in the airways was observed; 150 mL of saline solution were injected into the middle lobe, with 80 mL recovered; no acid-alcohol resistant bacilli (AARB) or r-RNA of MTC were found.

Finally, thoracentesis was performed. Thoracic ultrasonography showed a small pleural effusion layer, visible through only one intercostal space. Without the use of local anesthesia, a 20-gauge needle was introduced into the sixth intercostal space along the right posterior axillary line and only 45 mL of liquid was evacuated. Chemical–physical examination of pleural fluid showed that it was exudative, according to Light's criteria: pH 7.40; total protein 4.1 g/dL; lactate dehydrogenase (LDH) 2,524 units/L; and glucose 57 mg/dL. The microscopy result was negative for AARB, whereas that of PCR for r-RNA of MTC was positive.

Discussion Topic

Pulmonologist

The patient, who is a general physician, has probably been infected by one of her patients suffering from unrecognized active pulmonary tuberculosis.

Infectious disease specialist

The use of active agents against MTC, such as levofloxacin, together with glucocorticoids, provided a slight clinical improvement but delayed the diagnosis.

Pulmonologist

The positivity of anti-*Mycoplasma pneumoniae* IgM was a confounding factor. This misled us into thinking that we had found the right diagnosis.

Antituberculosis therapy was started with isoniazid, rifampin, pyrazinamide, and ethambutol, according to the World Health Organization (WHO) guidelines. The patient was discharged with the diagnosis of tuberculous pleural effusion.

The four-drug therapy was continued for 2 months, after which the patient returned for a scheduled follow-up visit to the clinic. The culture results, which had arrived by then, were positive for MTC, with good susceptibility to isoniazid, rifampin, pyrazinamide, and ethambutol.

A two-drug therapy (isoniazid and rifampin) was subsequently performed for an additional 4 months.

The patient received the antituberculosis therapy for a total of 6 months without any interruption.

Subsequently, chest radiography and chest CT showed resolution of the right pleural effusion (Figs. 8.3 and 8.4). Blood test results were normal as well. No further therapy was necessary.

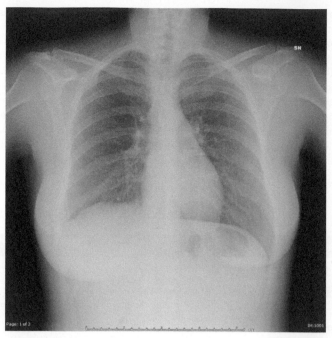

Fig. 8.3   Chest radiograph showing a resolution of the right pleural effusion with a sharp costophrenic angle.

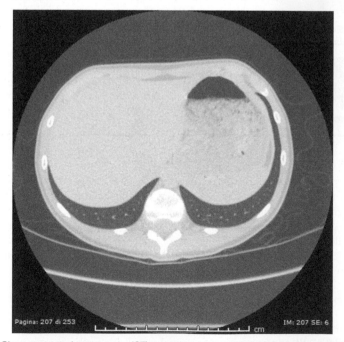

Fig. 8.4   Chest computed tomography (CT) scan showing a resolution of the right pleural effusion.

Focus On

Indications for Diagnostic Thoracentesis

Most individuals with newly identified pleural effusion should undergo diagnostic thoracentesis. The procedure consists of percutaneous insertion of a needle through the intercostal space with the aim of draining a variable quantity of pleural fluid. Thoracentesis may provide information on the macroscopic features of pleural fluid and helps identify the cause of pleural effusion. It is not indicated when the diagnosis is clinically certain (e.g., heart failure or recent surgery), unless there is fever, pleuritic chest pain, unilateral effusion, or considerable discrepancy in size of the pleural effusion on the left and right sides, echocardiography result inconsistent with heart failure, and lack of reduction in pleural effusion despite optimal fluid management. Diagnostic thoracentesis is usually avoided if the pleural effusion is less than 1 cm on lateral decubitus radiography, ultrasonography, or computed tomography.

Focus On

Chest Ultrasonography and Pleural Diseases

Chest ultrasonography is a very useful diagnostic tool for evaluation of pleural diseases. It is rapid, noninvasive, and can be performed at the patient's bedside. Pleural effusion is typically anechoic; however, the cause and chronicity of pleural effusion influence its physical characteristics and thus the ultrasonographic aspect. Moreover, chest ultrasonography can be used as a guide for improving the safety of interventional procedures, such as thoracentesis, chest tube insertion, and needle aspiration biopsy of pleural or subpleural lung masses.

Focus On

Tuberculous Pleural Effusion

Tuberculous pleural effusion (TPE) is one of the most common forms of extrapulmonary TB. In the United States and Europe, it occurs in approximately 5% of patients with *Mycobacterium tuberculosis* infection, whereas in some areas of Africa, up to 25% of patients with TB have pleural involvement, with a higher percentage in patients with human immunodeficiency virus (HIV) infection.

TPE usually presents as an acute illness with fever, cough, and pleuritic chest pain. Usually pleural fluid, which is an exudate, predominantly has lymphocytes. The diagnosis of tuberculous pleuritis requires the detection of *Mycobacterium tuberculosis* in pleural fluid or in pleural biopsy specimens (either by microscopy and/or culture) or the histological demonstration of caseating granulomas in the pleura along with acid-fast bacilli (AFB). Identification of adenosine deaminase (ADA) and interferon-γ in pleural fluid has been documented to be useful for the diagnosis of TPE. High ADA levels in lymphocyte-predominant exudate justify treatment initiation in patients with a high pretest probability.

Pleural involvement may occur in primary and postprimary (i.e. reactivated) TB. Until recently, TPE was thought to occur largely as the result of delayed hypersensitivity reactions. However, currently available culture media allows for culturing *Mycobacterium tuberculosis* from both pleural fluid and pleural tissue in more than two out three cases. More specifically, microscopy of pleural fluid can identify AFB in less than 10% of patients. Culture of pleural fluid on solid media has a sensitivity of 12% to 30%, whereas liquid culture media have sensitivity of up to 70%. Even in negative fluids studies, thoracoscopy often reveals extensive inflammatory granuloma formation and fibrin deposits, with unexpected recovery of abundant mycobacteria. Thus TPE is now believed to be the manifestation of direct paucibacillary mycobacterial infection of the pleural space, from contiguous lung lesions or lymphogenic or hematogenic spread, resulting in an immunological response.

LEARNING POINTS

- In patients with pleural effusion, an accurate assessment for risk of TB is always recommended.
- For patients with unilateral pleural effusion, diagnostic thoracentesis is recommended.
- Fluoroquinolones are effective against many mycobacterial species, including most strains of MTC.
- In patients unable to produce sputum specimens, *Mycobacterium tuberculosis* can be identified in gastric aspirate, bronchial washing, pleural fluid, urine, and cerebrospinal fluid specimens.
- Identification of genetic material in biological specimens with the use of PCR is a rapid and reliable test for the diagnosis of active TB.

Further Reading

1. Zhai K, Lu Y, Shi HZ. Tuberculous pleural effusion. *J Thorac Dis.* 2016;8(7):E486–E494.
2. Shaw JA, Irusen EM, Diacon AH, Koegelenberg CF. Pleural tuberculosis: a concise clinical review. *Clin Respir J.* 2018;12(5):1779–1786.
3. Vorster MJ, Allwood BW, Diacon AH, Koegelenberg CF. Tuberculous pleural effusions: advances and controversies. *J Thorac Dis.* 2015;7(6):981–991.
4. Horsburgh CR, Jr., Barry CE, 3rd, Lange C. Treatment of tuberculosis. *N Engl J Med.* 2015; 373(22):2149–2160.
5. Ruan SY, Chuang YC, Wang JY, et al. Revisiting tuberculous pleurisy: pleural fluid characteristics and diagnostic yield of mycobacterial culture in an endemic area. *Thorax.* 2012;67:822–827.
6. Porcel JM. Advances in the diagnosis of tuberculous pleuritis. *Ann Transl Med.* 2016;4(15):282.
7. Sorino C, Cappelletti T. Tuberculosis diagnostics: in vivo and in vitro techniques. In: Sorino C, ed. *Diagnostic Evaluation of the Respiratory System.* New Delhi: Jaypee Brothers Medical Publishers; 2017.

CHAPTER 9

Loculated Parapneumonic Pleural Effusion Treated With Intracavitary Urokinase

Alessandro Zanforlin ■ Claudio Sorino ■ Michele Mondoni

History of Present Illness

A 58-year-old man arrived at the emergency room with high fever, dyspnea, anorexia with loss of weight, weakness, and confusion.

Past Medical History

The patient was a current smoker of 15 to 20 cigarettes a day (40 pack-year). He had a history of long-term alcohol abuse, with consequent psychosis, ataxia, and fatty liver.

Physical Examination and Early Clinical Findings

The patient was alert but confused and disoriented. He was pale, had poor fat and muscle mass, and had a body mass index of 19 kg/m². Blood pressure was low (90/60 mm Hg). Arterial blood gas analyses in room air showed acute respiratory failure without hypercapnia: pH 7.42; partial pressure of oxygen (PaO₂ 54.3 mm Hg); partial pressure of carbon dioxide (PaCO₂) 41.6 mm Hg; and bicarbonate (HCO₃⁻) 24.5. Blood tests showed marked leukocytosis (37,000/μL) and high inflammation indexes (C-reactive protein (CRP) 324 mg/dL; procalcitonin 10.9 ng/mL).

Chest examination revealed absence of vesicular murmur in the lower field of left hemithorax. Rare fine crackles were appreciated in the middle and upper fields of the same side. No pathological findings were observed on the left hemithorax. No peripheral edema was present. Chest radiography performed in the emergency room showed multiple opacities, with tapering obtuse margins along the right lateral chest wall and at the right lung base, suggestive of loculated pleural effusion (Fig. 9.1). The patient was admitted to the internal medicine department.

Clinical Course

The patient was given supplemental 50% oxygen via a Venturi mask and intravenous fluids (continuous 0.9% saline at 60 mL/h). Empiric antibiotic therapy was started with oral levofloxacin 750 mg a day and intravenous piperacillin/tazobactam 4.5 g three times a day. Chest ultrasonography showed organized pleural effusion with multiple adhesions and loculations in lower-posterior, lateral, lower-anterior, and upper-anterior zones, with an underlying partially consolidated lung (Fig. 9.2, A and B). Despite the therapy, in the subsequent 72 hours, the patient showed persistent signs of dysventilation of the right lung and further episodes of fever.

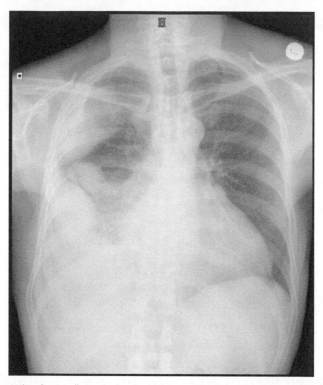

Fig. 9.1 Posteroanterior chest radiograph showing right opacities obscuring adjacent structures, suggestive of multiloculated right pleural effusion.

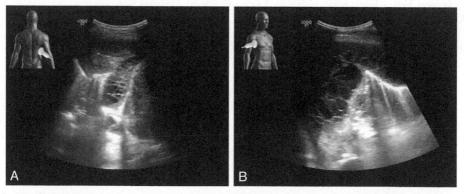

Fig. 9.2 (A and B) Chest ultrasonography (convex probe) images showing loculated pleural effusion with fibrin strands.

Discussion Topic

Internist

There is high clinical suspicion of pleural empyema. We need to evacuate the pleural fluid.

Discussion Topic—cont'd

Pulmonologist A

Certainly, it's complicated pleural effusion. Chest ultrasonography leaves no doubts. Empyema is defined as the presence of pus in the pleural cavity. So we can understand if that is the case just by extracting the pleural fluid.

Pulmonologist B

In both cases, the treatment does not differ. In the presence of such a thickly organized fibrin net, thoracentesis is not recommended. The placement of pleural drainage is mandatory.

Pulmonologist A

Even this could be insufficient to adequately clean the pleural cavity.

Internist

Do you think that thoracoscopy will be necessary?

Pulmonologist B

Early treatment by thoracoscopic debridement could improve the outcome of pleural empyema.

Thoracic surgeon

The patient is very weak and has poor hemodynamic conditions. Surgical thoracoscopy could be dangerous.

Pulmonologist A

Surely chest computed tomography (CT) can help choose the best approach.

Pulmonologist B

Ok, but let's not forget that a delay in surgery can cause subsequent need for more complex procedures, such as decortication.

Chest computed tomography (CT) (Fig. 9.3, A and B) showed multiloculated pleural fluid collections, confirming the ultrasonographic and radiographic findings. A 20-French (Fr) chest tube was inserted through the fifth intercostal space and connected to a water seal chamber. About

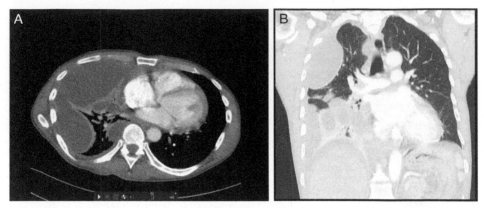

Fig. 9.3 Contrast-enhanced chest computed tomography (CT) scan showing right loculated pleural effusion. (A) Axial plane (soft tissue window). (B) Sagittal reconstruction (parenchymal window).

600 mL of dull yellow fluid highly suggestive for pus was drained (Fig. 9.4). Physical–chemical examination of pleural fluid was coherent with empyema: low pH (7.12); high level of lactate dehydrogenase (LDH; 2,200 units/L); and low glucose concentration (2.0 mmol/L). Microscopic examination for acid-fast bacilli (AFB) yielded a negative result.

Paracetamol 1 g three times a day was needed to control pain at the chest tube insertion site. After 2 days, the fever disappeared, and the inflammatory indices begun to decrease.

However, bedside ultrasonography showed incomplete lung expansion and persistence of extensive fibrin net with multiple pleural locules. The corresponding chest radiograph is shown in Fig. 9.5.

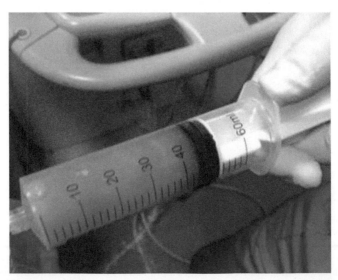

Fig. 9.4 A sample of extracted pleural fluid, which is purulent in appearance.

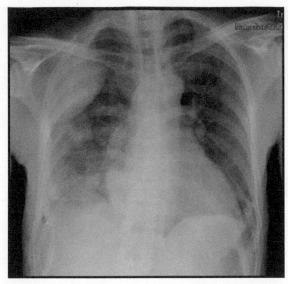

Fig. 9.5 Posteroanterior chest radiograph obtained soon after drainage positioning. A right loculated pleural effusion is still evident.

Discussion Topic

Pulmonologist A

How much pleural fluid came out of the drainage?

Internist

After the first 600 mL, about 150 mL per day.

Pulmonologist B

Ultrasonography shows persistence of extensive fibrin strands inside the pleural collections.

Internist

Yet I washed the pleural cavity with saline solution twice a day!

Pulmonologist A

Given the high risk of surgery, we can inject a fibrinolytic agent into the pleural cavity and evaluate the response.

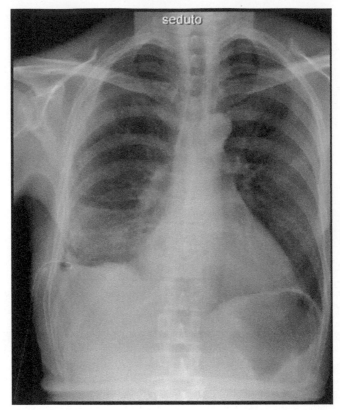

Fig. 9.6 Posteroanterior chest radiograph obtained 8 days after urokinase treatment. The upper right thorax transparency has improved. The chest tube is still in place, and a small amount of pleural effusion is still evident in the lower zone.

Cytological analysis of pleural fluid showed a negative result for malignant tumor cells. Cultures of pleural fluid and blood showed no growth of aerobic or anaerobic organisms.

Intracavitary treatment with urokinase was performed (100,000 units in 100 mL of saline, injected once a day through the chest drain and maintained within the pleural cavity for 3 hours). This was repeated on 5 consecutive days, resulting in progressive reduction of loculations and pleural effusion. Chest radiography was repeated after 4 and 8 days (Fig. 9.6). In the subsequent 48 hours, the chest drain was inactive, followed by its removal. Overall, the patient received antibiotic therapy for 20 days. Leucocytes and inflammation indices further decreased to normal values, and the patient was discharged.

Follow-Up and Outcomes

The sutures at the drainage insertion site were removed 3 weeks after their placement.

After 40 days, chest radiography and clinical examination demonstrated complete normalization of findings (Fig. 9.7).

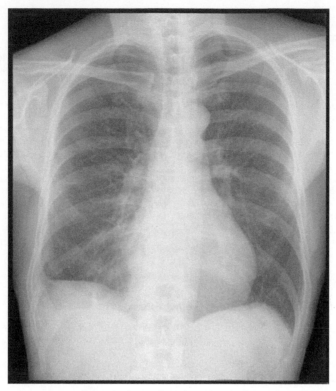

Fig. 9.7 Posteroanterior chest radiograph obtained 40 days after discharge. The right pleural effusion has almost completely resolved; minimal blunting of the costophrenic angle is recognizable.

Focus On

Chemical–Physical Examination of the Pleural Fluid

The mechanism of formation of pleural effusion affects the biochemical characteristics of the fluid. Chemical–physical examination is commonly used to distinguish pleural effusions into transudates and exudates.

Transudative effusions result from imbalances in hydrostatic and oncotic forces and have a low protein content (pleural/serum protein ratio ≤ 0.5) and low lactate dehydrogenase (LDH) content (LDH ≤ 200 units/L or pleural/serum LDH ratio ≤ 0.6). Heart failure and cirrhosis are the most common causes. They may also occur in nephrotic syndrome, atelectasis, peritoneal dialysis, constrictive pericarditis, superior vena cava obstruction, and urinothorax.

If the physical–chemical examination suggests that pleural fluid is of transudative nature, further diagnostic procedures are not required, and treatment of the underlying condition (e.g., diuretic therapy) usually reduces the pleural effusion.

Exudative effusions are caused by local factors that increase the permeability of the pleural surfaces and blood vessels, favoring the accumulation of pleural fluid. Pneumonia, malignancy, and thromboembolism account for most exudative effusions. They usually have a relatively high protein and LDH content (pleural/serum protein ratio > 0.5; LDH > 200 units/L or pleural/serum LDH ratio > 0.6).

Further pleural fluid analyses (cell counts and differential, glucose, adenosine deaminase, cytological analysis) are often useful to clarify the cause of exudative effusion.

Focus On

Parapneumonic Effusion and Empyema

A parapneumonic effusion (i.e., an effusion that forms in the pleural space adjacent to pneumonia) is usually an inflammatory exudate with predominance of polymorphonuclear leukocytes. An empyema (i.e. the presence of pus in the pleural space) is caused by bacterial invasion of the pleural space, which may complicate a simple parapneumonic effusion. In such a case, the pleural effusion is usually acidic, with pH less than 7.20 as a result of the increase in lactic acid production; it has high levels of LDH (> 1000 units/L) as a result of leukocyte death; and low glucose concentration (< 2.2 mmol/L) as a result of an increase in glucose metabolism. The above-mentioned factors constitute the biochemical criteria for pleural infection. Pleural fluid pH is the most useful index predicting the need for chest tube drainage and is highly recommended when the pH value is less than 7.2.

In patients with parapneumonic pleural effusions, the placement of a thoracic drainage tube is always indicated when pleural fluid consists of pus or when culture results are positive. It is also recommended if the effusion is loculated or is half the hemithorax or larger, if pH is less than 7.2, and if the pleura is thickened, as seen on contrast-enhanced CT (Table 9.1).

Focus On

Role of Fibrinolytics in Complicated Pleural Effusions

Complicated parapneumonic effusions (low pH, low glucose, high lactate dehydrogenase [LDH] or empyema [frank pus] fibrin) may create intrapleural locules that make fluid drainage and lung expansion difficult.

Intrapleural instillation of fibrinolytic drugs may help lyse fibrin adhesions, promote pleural drainage, and avoid surgery. Agents commonly used include streptokinase, urokinase, and recombinant tissue plasminogen activator (rtPA). After their introduction into the pleural cavity, the fibrinolytics are usually left to act, with the tube closed for about 3 hours.

The suggested dosages of the current fibrinolytics in use are as follows:
- Streptokinase: 250,000 units in 100 to 200 mL of saline, instilled once a day for up to 7 days (until drainage < 100 mL/day)
- Urokinase: 100,000 units in 100 mL of saline, instilled once a day for up to 3 days
- rtPA: 10 to 25 mg in 100 mL of saline, instilled twice daily for up to 3 days

Fibrinolytic drugs have negligible effects with regard to decreasing the viscosity of the empyema pus in contrast to agents that depolymerize DNA, such as human recombinant deoxyribonuclease (DNase). Clinical trials on concurrent administration of rtPA and DNase in patients with pleural infection suggested that it is relatively safe and effective. Given the high cost of therapy, it would be feasible to determine therapy on the basis of clinical and radiographic responses. A possible scheme of administration is as follows:
- rtPA 10 mg in 50 mL of saline
- DNase 5 mg in 50 mL of saline, followed by a 60-mL saline flush, administered twice daily up to a maximum of six doses over 3 days

TABLE 9.1 ■ A Possible System for Staging Parapneumonic Pleural Effusion With Indication for Procedures

Effusion Stage	Macroscopic Features	Microbiology	Chemistry	Procedure
Uncomplicated parapneumonic pleural effusion	Small-to-moderate free-flowing effusion (less than one-half hemithorax)	Negative culture and Gram staining	pH > 7.20 or glucose > 60 mg/dL	Thoracentesis (if pleural effusion > 10 mm)
Complicated parapneumonic pleural effusion	Large free-flowing effusion (≥ one-half hemithorax), or loculated effusion, or effusion with thickened parietal pleura	Positive culture or Gram staining	pH < 7.20 or glucose < 60 mg/dL	Drainage or thoracoscopy
Empyema		Frank pus	Tests not indicated	

LEARNING POINTS

- Protein-rich exudative effusion may form fibrin strands and multiple intrapleural loculations.
- Intrapleural instillation of fibrinolytics can help lyse fibrin adhesions, promote pleural drainage, and avoid surgery.
- Pleural fluid bacterial culture should be performed, and pH should be assessed if empyema is a concern.
- Video thoracoscopic debridement is a useful treatment option for loculated pleural empyema.
- Standard pleural fluid culture is negative in about 40% of empyema cases.

Further Reading

1. Light RW. Parapneumonic effusions and empyema. *Proc Am Thorac Soc*. 2006;3:75–80.
2. Altmann ES, Crossingham I, Wilson S, Davies HR. Intra-pleural fibrinolytic therapy versus placebo, or a different fibrinolytic agent, in the treatment of adult parapneumonic effusions and empyema. *Cochrane Database Syst Rev*. 2019;2019(10):CD002312.
3. Yu H. Management of pleural effusion, empyema, and lung abscess. *Semin Intervent Radiol*. 2011;28:75–86.
4. Abu-Daff S, Maziak DE, Alshehab D, et al. Intrapleural fibrinolytic therapy (IPFT) in loculated pleural effusions—analysis of predictors for failure of therapy and bleeding: a cohort study. *BMJ Open*. 2013;3:e001887.
5. Rosenstengel A. Pleural infection-current diagnosis and management. *J Thorac Dis*. 2012;4(2):186–193.
6. Menzies SM, Rahman NM, Wrightson JM, et al. Blood culture bottle culture of pleural fluid in pleural infection. *Thorax*. 2011;66(8):658–662.
7. Sheikh HE, Abd Rabboh MM. Chest ultrasound in the evaluation of complicated pneumonia in the ICU patients: can be viable alternative to CT? *Egypt J Radiol Nucl Med*. 2014;45:325–331.
8. Rahman NM, Kahan BC, Miller RF, et al. A clinical score (RAPID) to identify those at risk for poor outcome at presentation in patients with pleural infection. *Chest*. 2014;145:848–855.

CHAPTER 10

Primary Pleural Empyema in a Hemodialysis Patient With Catheter-Related Bloodstream Infection

Claudio Sorino ▪ Fabio Pirracchio ▪ Sergio Agati ▪ Abdul Hamid Alraiyes

History of Present Illness

An 81-year-old woman arrived in the emergency room (ER) because of progressive fatigue for 1 week, with worsening dyspnea and decreased urine output. Before that ER visit, the general practitioner had placed the patient on oral furosemide, with no improvement of symptoms. Two weeks earlier, the patient had also received a course of amoxicillin/clavulanic acid for urinary tract infection.

Past Medical History

The patient, who was a never-smoker, had a history of arterial hypertension, hypothyroidism, and ischemic heart disease. Eight years earlier, she had undergone coronary angiography with angioplasty and stent placement for myocardial infarction. The procedure was complicated by subacute occlusion of the superficial femoral artery. Two years before her current presentation, she had also undergone gastrectomy with esophagojejunostomy for gastric adenocarcinoma. Her home medication list included amlodipine, levothyroxine, acetylsalicylic acid, and furosemide.

Physical Examination and Early Clinical Findings

On presentation, the patient was pale, dyspneic, and tachycardic. She was anuric for the past 24 hours, did not have any vomiting or diarrhea, and did not take nonsteroidal anti-inflammatory drugs recently. Blood pressure was 115/80 mm Hg. Upon auscultation, the breath sounds were found to be slightly reduced, mainly at the bases. Physical examination findings of the abdomen were unremarkable. Blood tests showed severe renal failure (serum creatinine 11.99 mg/dL, urea 305 mg/dL); hyperkalemia (potassium 6.4 mEq/L), mild leukocytosis (white blood cell [WBC] count 10,820/mm^3); severe microcytic anemia (hemoglobin [Hb] 5.8 g/dL, mean corpuscular volume 74 fL; normal range 80–95 fL), and high brain-type natriuretic peptide (proBNP 32,500 pg/mL; values > 400 pg/mL strongly suggestive of ventricular dysfunction). The platelet count was 125,000 cells/μL, and the international normalized ratio (INR) was 1.09.

Although oxygen saturation on pulse oximetry (SpO$_2$) was 93% while the patient was breathing room air, arterial blood gas analyses (ABG) analyses showed hypoxemic respiratory failure with a partial pressure of oxygen (PaO$_2$) of 53 mm Hg.

Abdominal ultrasonography demonstrated a minimal amount of perihepatic intraperitoneal fluid. The sizes of both kidneys were slightly reduced (pole-to-pole length 10 and 9 cm for the

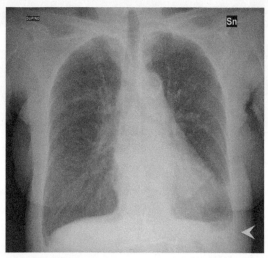

Fig. 10.1 Portable chest radiograph obtained at admission (anteroposterior, supine position) showing a small left pleural effusion *(arrowhead)*.

left and right kidneys, respectively). Hydronephrosis and kidney stones were not observed. Chest ultrasonography revealed mild bilateral pleural effusion, pulmonary vertical artifacts, and large lower vena cava with inspiratory collapse less than 50%.

Chest radiography confirmed small left pleural effusion, with no evident lung parenchymal lesions (Fig. 10.1).

Discussion Topic

ER doctor A

Arterial oxygen is lower than I expected. Do you think that a mixture of venous and arterial blood occurred during puncturing for the arterial blood gas (ABG) analysis?

ER doctor B

No, patients with anemia may have sufficient SpO_2 levels but a low arterial partial pressure of oxygen (PaO_2). Hemoglobin (Hb) is well saturated, but it is the total Hb quantity that is reduced! Thus the oxygen carried to the tissues will also be scarce.

Nephrologist

She needs a red blood cell transfusion quickly and hemodialysis. I'll place a femoral central venous catheter (CVC).

ER doctor A

Why do you prefer the femoral access? There, the catheter has an increased risk of infection.

Discussion Topic—cont'd

Nephrologist

During emergencies, CVC can be placed quickly in the femoral vein. The immediate complication rate is lower than placement in the internal jugular or subclavian veins.

ER doctor B

I agree. There's no risk of pneumothorax, and accidental arterial puncture can be easily addressed with direct pressure. Moreover, placement of a CVC in the femoral vein is more comfortable in individuals with fluid overload because patients don't need to be completely supine.

ER doctor A

We should also understand why anemia developed in this patient.

ER doctor B

Chronic kidney disease is a possible cause. We should consider erythropoietin supplementation.

Nephrologist

Anemia in chronic kidney disease (CKD) is usually normocytic. However, the patient has few and small red blood cells. She could have had blood loss, too. Let's not forget that she regularly takes an antiplatelet!

ER doctor B

The search for fecal occult blood will be useful. Moreover, we should rule out hemolysis.

Nephrologist

I'll order serum iron and transferrin tests, too. Erythropoietin doesn't work if iron blood levels and transferrin saturation are low.

Clinical Course

A central venous catheter was placed in the right deep femoral vein under ultrasound guidance. The patient immediately underwent red blood cell transfusion and diuretic therapy; then she was admitted to the nephrology department, where hemodialysis was initiated.

Further investigation showed anti–glomerular basement membrane (GBM) antibodies in serum and high-titer perinuclear antineutrophil cytoplasmic antibodies (p-ANCA). Therefore immuno-suppression was initiated with high-dose systemic corticosteroids (intravenous methylprednisolone

500 mg/day for 3 days, followed by oral prednisone 1 mg/kg/day) and oral cyclophosphamide 2 mg/kg/day. After correction of anemia and electrolyte balance, the patient underwent ultrasound-guided percutaneous kidney biopsy. Histological examination showed crescentic glomerulonephritis with extensive signs of chronic vasculitis. Serum iron was 32 μg/dL (normal range 60–170 μg/dL), whereas transferrin was 330 mg/dL (normal range 250–350 μg/dL), with transferrin saturation 7% (normal range for women 15%–50%). Administration of intravenous iron and subcutaneous erythropoietin was initiated. The test for fecal occult blood showed a positive result. Esophagogastroduodenoscopy did not show any source of bleeding. The patient declined colonoscopy.

Five days after admission, renal function and urine output had not improved, and the patient was placed on three-times–weekly hemodialysis.

During hospitalization, a fever with and chills occurred, and systemic inflammation markers increased. The highest values of C-reactive protein (CRP) and procalcitonin (PCT) were 298 mg/L and 4.97 ng/mL, respectively. The patient also complained of shortness of breath, and high-flow oxygen (FiO_2; 40% via a Venturi mask) supplement was necessary to obtain sufficient oxygen saturation (SpO_2).

Discussion Topic

Nephrologist

The patient has signs of sepsis and respiratory symptoms! She probably has a lower respiratory tract infection.

Internist

This is a possibility. On auscultation, I found a strong reduction in respiratory sounds and dullness in the middle and lower left fields. Oxygen saturation (SpO_2) was 85%, I gave oxygen supplement with fraction of inspired oxygen (FiO_2) 40% via a Venturi mask to get SpO_2 of 93%.

Nephrologist

We can introduce empirical antibiotic therapy for nosocomial pneumonia, with gram-negative coverage. However, a chest radiography or ultrasonography will be useful to confirm this.

Internist

I would also add coverage for methicillin-resistant *Staphylococcus aureus.*
She could have septicemia, too. Before starting the antibiotic, blood culture specimens need to be collected.

Nephrologist

We have no other biological samples to examine. She has no sputum and is anuric.

Internist

It's crucial to see if the patient's condition worsens to septic shock. We will monitor blood pressure and vital signs (body temperature, pulse rate, respiration rate).

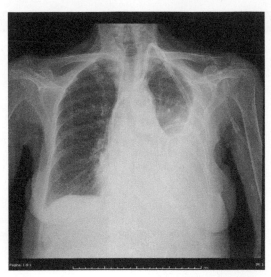

Fig. 10.2   Chest radiograph (anteroposterior, sitting position) showing a significant increase in left pleural effusion.

Empirical antibiotic therapy was undertaken on the basis of the assumption that the patient could have a hospital-acquired lower respiratory tract infection with sepsis. Antibiotics active against methicillin-resistant *Staphylococcus aureus* (MRSA), gram-negative bacteria, and *Pseudomonas aeruginosa* were included: piperacillin/tazobactam 2.25 g intravenous (IV) every 8 hours and vancomycin, at a loading dose of 20 mg/kg IV and maintenance doses of 10 mg/kg IV after each dialysis. After 24 hours, the attending physicians were notified that blood culture results were positive for gram-positive cocci.

The central catheter was removed, and a tunneled hemodialysis catheter was placed in the left internal jugular vein (because of stenosis of the right internal jugular vein, usually preferred site). Definitive blood culture results revealed the growth of methicillin-sensitive *Staphylococcus aureus* (MSSA); thus vancomycin administration was stopped.

Despite optimization of fluid management, low-grade fever and respiratory failure persisted, and chest radiography revealed an increase in the left pleural effusion (Fig. 10.2). A pulmonologist was consulted, and he ordered thoracic ultrasonography, which showed that the pleural effusion had an initial tendency to fibrinous organization (Fig. 10.3).

Discussion Topic

Nephrologist

Can the pleural effusion be linked to the presence of autoimmune vasculitis?

Pulmonologist

I don't think so. Anti–glomerular basement membrane (GBM) antibodies are present in Goodpasture syndrome. It usually affects the lung parenchyma and presents as alveolar hemorrhage, whereas the pleura is not commonly involved.

Continued

Discussion Topic—cont'd

Nephrologist

So could it be a parapneumonic effusion?

Pulmonologist

It is certainly a complicated pleural effusion, and the fluid must be removed and analyzed. Rapid appearance of fibrin is usually the expression of intense inflammation within the pleural cavity.

Nephrologist

Probably she's debilitated, and the efficiency of her immune system is reduced. Not sure that the systemic corticosteroid also played a role, because the treatment was only recently started.

Pulmonologist

Contrast computed tomography (CT) of the chest would be helpful. Can the patient undergo it?

Nephrologist

Sure. We'll schedule a dialysis session immediately after it. Echocardiography will also be useful to rule out the presence of valvular vegetations.

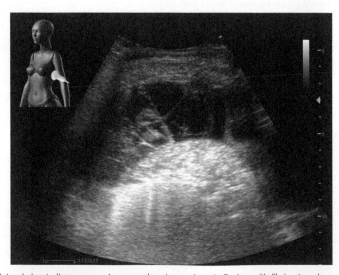

Fig. 10.3 Left lateral chest ultrasonography scan showing a pleural effusion with fibrin strands and floating debris.

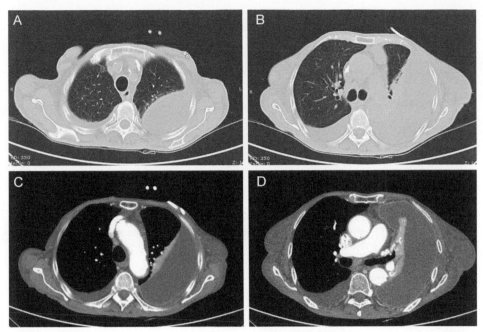

Fig. 10.4 Chest computed tomography (CT) scan (A, B: lung window; C, D: mediastinal window) showing a large area of left pleural effusion with atelectasis of the adjacent lung parenchyma and a small area of contralateral pleural effusion.

High-resolution computed tomography (CT) of the chest with contrast medium was promptly performed. This confirmed a large area of left pleural effusion that compressed the adjacent pulmonary parenchyma. No frank pneumonia was present, and a small area of contralateral pleural effusion was also found (Fig. 10.4).

Discussion Topic

Nephrologist

The lung consolidation seems to be minor, and the patient has septicemia. Could the patient have developed a pleural infection secondary to bacteremia?

Pulmonologist

It's not common but possible. Some call it *primary empyema*. The treatment for it does not differ from that for an infection developed by contiguity and includes appropriate antibiotic therapy and prompt evacuation of the pleural fluid.

Pulmonologist 2

It is important to place a pleural drain as soon as possible. A delay may lead to a further organization of the space and worsen the outcome.

Continued

Nephrologist

The patient is very weak. Is thoracentesis not enough?

Pulmonologist

It would be a fallback. It would not ensure the complete evacuation of the pleural effusion, nor would it allow for washing the pleural cavity.

Pulmonologist 2

I agree. Given the appearance on ultrasonography, a chest tube is strongly recommended. Furthermore, I would avoid a small-bore drain, to reduce the risk of its becoming blocked by fibrin or clots.

Both platelet count and INR were adequate for pleural drainage. Under local anesthesia and ultrasound guidance, a 20-Fr chest tube was placed, resulting in prompt evacuation of 1500 mL of turbid pleural fluid. A further 450 mL of pleural fluid was evacuated about 1 hour later, then approximately 100 mL/day came out for 2 days.

The chemical–physical examination of this fluid was indicative of exudate and highly suggestive of empyema: leukocytes were more than four times higher than the upper limit of normal (4337 cells/mL, polymorphonuclear leukocytes 89%), LDH was very high (3243 U/L), and pH and glucose were low (7.19 and 47 g/dL, respectively).

Postprocedure chest radiography and ultrasonography showed residual organized pleural effusion with fibrin septa in the costodiaphragmatic recess (Figs. 10.5 and 10.6).

Consequently, urokinase was instilled in the pleural cavity through drainage (100,000 units in 100 mL of saline per day, for 3 consecutive days). At the same time, the patient was instructed to perform inspiratory and expiratory exercises by using an incentive spirometer to help chest expansion and assist in drainage of fluid. A further 500 mL of pleural fluid was drained off in 3 days, and then the flow rate of the pleural drainage progressively diminished and stopped in a few days. Chest radiography and ultrasonography confirmed resolution of the left pleural effusion, and blood tests showed the near normalization of systemic inflammatory markers (CRP 12.1 mg/L; PCT 0.93 ng/mL). Therefore the chest tube was removed. The pleural fluid cytological examination did not show malignant tumor cells, and culture yielded negative results. Echocardiography did not demonstrate any valvular vegetation.

Recommended Therapy and Further Indications at Discharge

The patient was discharged in stable clinical condition, without evidence of respiratory failure. She was advised to perform chest physiotherapy at home twice daily for a week and to continue taking oral cyclophosphamide and prednisone. Hemodialysis treatment was scheduled to be provided three times a week at the nephrology center.

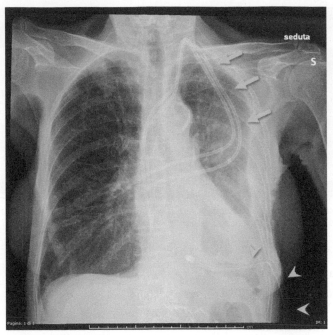

Fig. 10.5 Chest radiograph (anteroposterior, sitting position) obtained after the placement of a chest tube *(arrowheads)* showing a reduction in the left pleural effusion. The tunneled hemodialysis catheter with insertion in the left jugular vein is also evident *(arrows)*.

Follow-Up and Outcomes

One month after discharge, chest CT showed a normally expanding left lung with very small organized pleural effusion. In the left lower lobe, there were minimal fibrotic lines and bronchiectasis (Fig. 10.7). Renal damage was very extensive and resulted in end-stage kidney disease; however, there was no evidence of extrarenal involvement of vasculitis. Therefore cyclophosphamide was stopped, and prednisone was rapidly tapered.

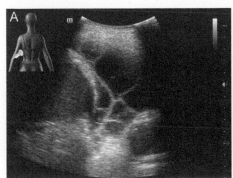
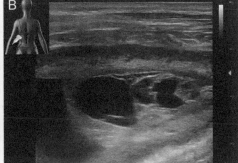

Fig. 10.6 Chest ultrasonography scan obtained after chest tube placement (A: convex probe; B: linear probe). A residual organized pleural effusion is evident, with fibrin septa inside the anechoic pleural space in the costodiaphragmatic recess.

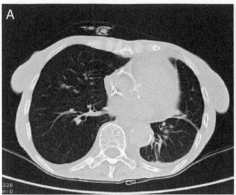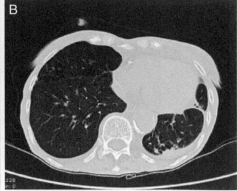

Fig. 10.7   A and B, Chest computed tomography (CT) scan after discharge (lung window) showing the residual aspects of a conservatively treated empyema.

Focus On

Routes and Mechanism of Pleural Infections

Most pleural space infections occur as a complication of community-acquired or hospital-acquired pneumonia. A proportion of pleural space infection results from iatrogenic causes. It is also known that pleural infection may occasionally develop (< 5%) without pneumonia or penetrating injury across the parietal pleura. When empyema develops in the absence of underlying radiographic evidence of pneumonia or other obvious cause, it is called *primary empyema*. This can occur during bacteremia, mainly caused by *Staphylococcus aureus* and invasive group A streptococcal infections. Table 10.1 lists the main causes and relevant mechanisms of pleural infection.

TABLE 10.1 ■ **Possible Mechanism and Causes of Pleural Infection**

Mechanisms	Causes
Transpleural translocation from adjacent consolidated lung	Pulmonary infection, mainly by oral anaerobes
Visceral pleural defects or fistulae	Infiltrating lung cancer
	Radiation therapy
	Postoperative complications (e.g., bronchial stump dehiscence)
	Necrotizing pneumonia, tuberculosis, fungal infections
Hematogenous spread	Bacteremia
	Uncertain role of pre-existing pleural effusion
Penetrating injury across pleura	Thoracic trauma
	Iatrogenic factors (invasive pleuropulmonary procedures)
Spread from mediastinum	Esophageal injury
	Postoperative factors
Transdiaphragmatic translocation	Intra-abdominal infections/ peritonitis (role of alcoholic cirrhosis)

Focus On

Patient Preparation Before Chest Tube Placement

Except in emergency conditions, before placement of a pleural drain, the patient should be informed about the potential risks and benefits of the procedure and should be asked to provide informed consent.

Nonurgent procedures should be postponed if the international normalized ratio (INR) is higher than 1.5 or the platelet count is less than 50,000 cells/mm³. Local anesthesia is usually sufficient for pain control, usually performed by infiltrating the skin, subcutaneous tissue, and parietal pleura with 1% to 2% mepivacaine or 1% to 2% lidocaine (no more than 20 mL, to avoid central nervous system effects, such as drowsiness, confusion, and convulsions, or cardiovascular effects, such as hypotension and arrhythmias). Conscious sedation may be considered when inserting large-bore tubes in anxious or agitated individuals. Commonly used drugs include intravenous opioids (e.g., fentanyl 25–50 mcg over 2 minutes or morphine 2–5 mg over 5 minutes) and/or benzodiazepines (e.g., midazolam 1–5 mg or diazepam 2–5 mg). Because respiratory depression is a possible side effect of sedatives, oxygen saturation should be continuously monitored, and reversing agents should be immediately accessible (naloxone for opioids; flumazenil for benzodiazepines).

Chest tube insertion is a fully aseptic technique. Routine administration of prophylactic antibiotics is recommended only in patients with penetrating chest injuries.

The ideal site of chest tube insertion is the fourth to fifth intercostal space in the midaxillary line. The patient should be placed in the supine position and slightly rotated, with the ipsilateral arm behind the head. In the case of posterior loculated fluid collection, the patient can remain in the seated position. In the case of apical or anterior pneumothorax, the second intercostal space in the midclavicular line can be an alternative site. In this case, the patient can simply lie in the supine position. A common insertion method is the so-called free-hand technique, where the physician marks the entry point under ultrasound guidance and inserts the tube immediately thereafter. A linear probe and color-Doppler function may help detect the intercostal vessels.

Focus On

Acute Phase Reactants and Markers of Bacterial Infections

Acute phase reactants (APRs) are different plasma proteins used as biomarkers of the immune response. Despite their variability in the course of trauma, cancer, or autoimmune disorders, APRs are important for the diagnosis and management of infectious diseases. C-reactive protein (CRP) and procalcitonin (PCT) are the most used APRs for the evaluation of bacterial pulmonary infections (Fig. 10.8). CRP normal serum concentration is usually lower than 10 mg/L. After the onset of an inflammatory process, CRP increases within 4 to 8 hours and reaches a peak within 2 to 3 days. CRP level greater than 100 mg/L is a sign of severe bacterial infection. In intensive care units, such values have good sensitivity and specificity (both near 90%) for the detection of ventilator-associated pneumonia. Monitoring CRP is an important measure for the quick definition and strict management of antibiotic therapy.

PCT is a valid biomarker of sepsis and systemic or localized bacterial infections, especially pneumonia. Normal serum PCT concentration in healthy humans is very low (< 0.1 ng/L). After a triggering event, PCT starts to increase faster than CRP. It becomes detectable within 2 to 4 hours and peaks after 12 to 24 hours. PCT serum concentration lower than 0.25 ng/L rules out the bacterial infection if other clinical signs are absent; instead, when PCT level is over 0.5 ng/L, the prescription of antibiotic therapy is strictly recommended.

Although no threshold perfectly discriminates among pathogens, median PCT concentration during infections by viruses is lower (0.09 ng/mL) than those of atypical bacteria (0.20 ng/mL) and typical bacteria (2.5 ng/mL).

Interpretation of APRs levels requires more care in patients with renal disease. Although CRP values are higher than normal in renal impairment, PCT is not significantly affected by renal diseases.

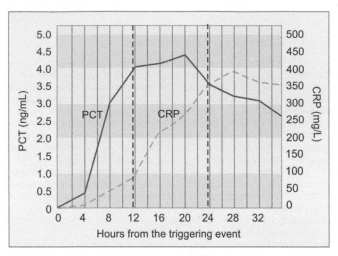

Fig. 10.8 Trends in blood levels of cross-reactive protein (CRP) and procalcitonin (PCT) after a major acute inflammatory stimulus. (Adapted from Magrì D, Oliviero G, Milani G, Sorino C. Clinical utility and interpretation of laboratory tests in respiratory medicine. In: Sorino C, ed. *Diagnostic Evaluation of the Respiratory System.* New Delhi: Jaypee Brothers Medical Publishers Ltd; 2017.)

LEARNING POINTS

- Although uncommon, a pleural infection can develop through the hematogenous route.
- Pleural empyema can result in high local inflammation with a rapid formation of fibrin and loculations in the pleural cavity.
- Chest ultrasonography is one of the most useful tools to assess the presence of complicated pleural effusion and evaluate the need for invasive procedures.
- Early intrapleural instillation of fibrinolytics can lead to the lysis of fibrin septa.
- Serum PCT is a good biomarker of bacterial infections and sepsis, especially pneumonia.
- After a triggering event, the PCT level starts to increase faster compared with that of CRP.

Further Reading

1. Semenkovich TR, Olsen MA, Puri V, Meyers BF, Kozower BD. Current state of empyema management. *Ann Thorac Surg.* 2018;105(6):1589–1596.
2. Porcel JM. Chest tube drainage of the pleural space: a concise review for pulmonologists. *Tuberc Respir Dis (Seoul).* 2018;81(2):106–115.
3. Greco A, Rizzo MI, De Virgilio A, et al. Goodpasture's syndrome: a clinical update. *Autoimmun Rev.* 2015;14(3):246–253.
4. Markanday A. Acute phase reactants in infections: evidence-based review and a guide for clinicians. *Open Forum Infect Dis.* 2015;2(3):ofv098.
5. Magrì D, Oliviero G, Milani G, Sorino C. Clinical utility and interpretation of laboratory tests in respiratory medicine. In: Sorino C, ed. *Diagnostic Evaluation of the Respiratory System.* New Delhi: Jaypee Brothers Medical Publishers Ltd; 2017:28–40.
6. Panichi V, Migliori M, De Pietro S, et al. C reactive protein in patients with chronic renal diseases. *Ren Fail.* 2001;23(3-4):551–562.
7. Corcoran JP, Wrightson JM, Belcher E, et al. Pleural infection: past, present, and future directions. *Lancet Respir Med.* 2015;3(7):563–577.
8. Yunt ZX, Frankel SK, Brown KK. Diagnosis and management of pulmonary vasculitis. *Ther Adv Respir Dis.* 2012;6(6):375–390.
9. Lu XL, Xiao ZH, Yang MY, Zhu YM. Diagnostic value of serum procalcitonin in patients with chronic renal insufficiency: a systematic review and meta-analysis. *Nephrol Dial Transplant.* 2012;28(1):122–129.

CHAPTER 11

Pyopneumothorax in Necrotizing Pneumonia With Bronchopleural Fistula

Giampietro Marchetti ■ Claudio Sorino ■ Stefano Negri ■ Valentina Pinelli

History of Present Illness

A 50-year-old Caucasian man presented to the emergency room with fever of 7 days' duration, shortness of breath, palpitations, and occasional cough with reddish brown, blood-stained sputum. He had been taking paracetamol, as needed. Chest radiography revealed abundant right hydropneumothorax (Fig. 11.1).

Past Medical History

The patient was a bartender, a current smoker of about 20 cigarettes a day (30 pack-year), with a history of alcohol abuse and fatty liver. He had undergone tonsillectomy in childhood.

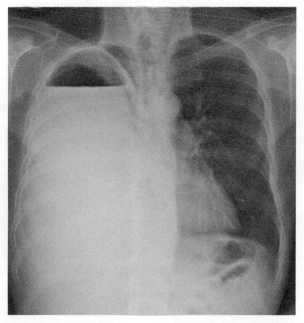

Fig. 11.1 Posteroanterior chest radiograph showing a large right hydropneumothorax, without evident mediastinal shift.

Physical Examination and Early Clinical Findings

The patient was alert, breathless at rest, and febrile (body temperature 38.4° C [101.12° F]). He had tachyarrhythmia, with heart rate 150 beats/min, and respiratory failure, with oxygen saturation measured by pulse oximetry (SpO_2) of 87% on room air. Respiratory rate was 25 breaths/min, and blood pressure was 170/85 mm Hg. Physical examination revealed absence of breath sounds to the right hemithorax. No pallor, clubbing, and peripheral edema were observed. Electrocardiography (ECG) revealed atrial fibrillation, with a high mean ventricular response.

Promptly 50% oxygen supplement was given via a Venturi mask. Arterial blood gas (ABG) analysis with this supplement resulted in sufficient correction of the partial pressure of oxygen (PaO_2 75 mm Hg); normal partial pressure of carbon dioxide ($PaCO_2$ 38 mm Hg); normal blood pH (7.39); and a slight increase in lactate (1.9 mmol/L). To reduce heart rate, a beta-blocker (metoprolol 5 mg intravenously over 5 minutes) was given, followed by a calcium channel blocker (diltiazem 20 mg intravenously over 2 minutes). Paracetamol 1 g was also administrated intravenously for the fever.

Blood tests showed elevated white blood cell (WBC) count (16,400 cells/mm^3) and high inflammatory indices (C-reactive protein [CRP] 234 mg/L). Hemoglobin was 12.7 g/dL, the platelet count was 122,000 cells/μL, and the international normalized ratio (INR) was 1.09. An anticoagulant (subcutaneous enoxaparin 6000 units, corresponding to 100 units anti-Xa activity/kg bodyweight, twice daily) and a broad-spectrum antibiotic (intravenous piperacillin/tazobactam 4 g/0.5 g, three times a day) were started as well. Blood cultures were performed.

After the initial treatment, heart rate dropped to around 100 beats/min. Chest ultrasonography showed pleural fluid that was not uniformly anechoic, with numerous floating hyperechoic pinpoints suggestive of empyemic hydropneumothorax (Fig. 11.2). Cardiac ultrasonography showed no abnormalities except for minimal mitral regurgitation. The ejection fraction of the left ventricle was normal (60%), and estimated systolic pulmonary pressure was not increased (30 mm Hg). There was no pericardial effusion.

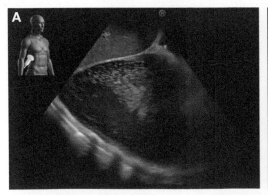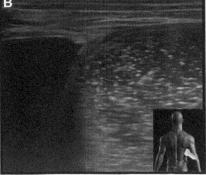

Fig. 11.2   Chest ultrasonography images (A: convex probe; B: linear probe) showing nonuniformly anechoic pleural fluid with numerous hyperechoic pinpoints (suspended microbubble sign) suggestive of empyemic hydropneumothorax (pyopneumothorax). The diaphragm was flattened and not very mobile.

Discussion topic

ER doctor

The patient has an hydropneumothorax and signs of sepsis. These probably triggered atrial fibrillation.

Pulmonologist

He's likely to have an alveolar-plural or a bronchopleural fistula, through which air and fluid passed into the pleural cavity.

ER doctor

Isn't that a complication of pneumonectomy or other pulmonary resection?

Pulmonologist

This is often the case. However, a bronchopleural fistula may also be due to other causes, such as pulmonary infection causing necrosis. Ultrasonography appearance suggest it, too.

ER doctor

Pleural effusion must be urgently evacuated by thoracentesis or drainage, right?

Pulmonologist

Given its large amount, I would place a chest tube.

Thoracic surgeon

The contemporary presence of fluid and air collections could require two drainages, one in the lower thorax, one in the upper.

Pulmonologist

It isn't a tension hydropneumothorax. Let's start with one tube in the lower thorax and see what happens.

Continued

Discussion Topic—cont'd

Thoracic surgeon

Okay. It's very likely that the patient has an empyema, so I'd place a large-bore drainage.

ER doctor

Enoxaparin was already administered, isn't it better to use a small-bore tube to decrease the bleeding risk?

Thoracic surgeon

Purulent fluid usually is very thick and corpuscular. Continuous washing will be necessary to clean the pleural cavity. I fear that a small-bore tube is inappropriate for this and would increase the risk of further chest tube placement or more invasive procedures.

ER doctor

We can administer Protamine sulfate to reverse the effects of enoxaparin.

Pulmonologist

Protamine sulfate use is not without risk. It is specifically indicated in heparin or LMWH overdose. Our patient has no evident bleeding, is hemodynamically stable, and mediastinum is not displaced. I would wait for the elimination of enoxaparin from the body before chest tube placement.

ER doctor

Ideally we should stop enoxaparin 24 hours before an invasive procedure.

Thoracic surgeon

I would not leave that effusion in the pleural cavity any longer. The patient could develop septic shock.

Pulmonologist

Our patient received only 6000 units of enoxaparin that has an half-life of 4.5 hours after a single dose, 7 hours after repeated dosing. I believe that the discontinuation of LMWH for 10–12 hours before the procedure is an acceptable compromise.

The patient received information regarding the insertion of a chest tube, and he gave his consent for the procedure. The thoracic surgeon waited 12 hours after enoxaparin administration. With the use of a small-gauge needle, the surgeon injected a local anesthetic (20 mL of lidocaine 200 mg/mL) into the fifth right intercostal space along the midaxillary line. Then a 2.5-cm incision was made along the superior edge of the inferior rib. A curved clamp was used to bluntly dissect through the subcutaneous tissues. Then a 24-French (Fr) pleural drainage was introduced by using the trocar technique. Abundant, creamy, foul-smelling pus (about 1500 mL) flowed out from the pleural space upon entry, together with many air bubbles. The drained pus was sent for microbiological tests. The patient experienced rapid subjective improvement and partial reappearance of breath sounds in the right hemithorax. Subsequently the patient was admitted to the pulmonology department.

Clinical Course

As recommended by the cardiologist, the patient received oral digoxin 0.125 mg once a day, oral diltiazem 60 mg twice daily, and subcutaneous enoxaparin 6000 units twice daily.

The pleural cavity was washed with saline two times daily through the double lumen thoracic drain. In about 36 hours, the fever disappeared, and the respiratory symptoms improved. In 48 hours, greater than 3000 mL of fluid was evacuated.

The chemical-physical examination of the pleural fluid was consistent with the diagnosis of empyema: low pH (7.17), low glucose concentration (30 mg/dL [1.66 mmol/L]), and high LDH levels (1800 units/L).

The microbiologist warned the physicians regarding the gram-positive cocci found in pleural fluid cultures, subsequently defined as colonies of methicillin-resistant *Staphylococcus aureus* (MRSA). Parenteral vancomycin 500 mg four times a day was added. In the following days, vancomycin trough concentrations at steady state were adequate ($\geq$ 15 µg/mL). Blood culture results were negative.

Chest radiography performed 1 week after pleural drain placement showed persistence of hydropneumothorax and incomplete expansion of the right lung (Fig. 11.3).

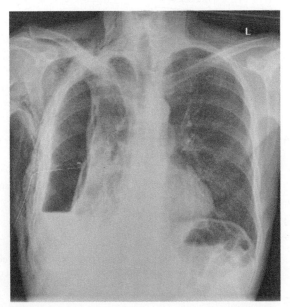

Fig. 11.3 Posteroanterior chest radiograph, obtained 1 week after chest tube placement, showing right hydropneumothorax with evident air–fluid level and partial lung collapse.

After 14 days of antibiotic therapy, the inflammatory indices became normal. With coughing, no further liquid, but only sporadic air, flowed from the pleural drainage. However, chest CT showed incomplete expansion of the right lung with persistence of pneumothorax and a small amount of fluid at the bottom of the pleural cavity. It also documented irregular lung hyperdensity, which, in correspondence with the apical segment of the right upper lobe, had an excavated area about 2 cm in diameter. This appeared to communicate with the pleural cavity through a thin through (Fig. 11.4).

Discussion Topic

Pulmonologist A

The lung did not expand adequately despite pleural drainage! What do you think about applying suction or the patient started on breathing exercises?

Thoracic surgeon

I fear that neither will benefit the patient. He seems to have a trapped lung and may require surgery.

Pulmonologist A

Actually, trapped lung is a chronic entity, which remains stable over time. It develops when the pleural inflammation lasts for a long time causing a mesothelial cells reaction that can lead to fibrosis. If the process that traps the lung is still active, we should call it *lung entrapment.*

Pulmonologist B

I agree. If the onset of symptoms is recent, I doubt that it has already resulted in trapped lung.

Pulmonologist A

Could it be useful to instill a fibrinolytic, such as urokinase, into the pleural cavity?

Pulmonologist B

No, I think, because I didn't see septa or loculations on ultrasonography. In my opinion, the lung will expand slowly. It just needs more time.

Pulmonologist C

The computed tomography (CT) scan is not clear. There's probably a bronchopleural fistula, which explains the persistent air in the pleural cavity. It can be a complication of necrotizing pneumonia.

Discussion Topic—cont'd

Pulmonologist A

What if the lung had pre-existing disease? The lung hyperdensity could be cancer, for example, complicated by empyema.

Pulmonologist C

I agree, malignancy is a possible cause of a peripheral fistula. I think it would be useful to perform bronchoscopy. This could also verify if the airways have a catarrhal footprint, which is another condition that can hinder lung expansion.

Pulmonologist B

We will certainly perform bronchoscopy. However, the lung may not have pre-existing disease. Empyema can trap the lung even in 15 to 20 days. We should also explore the pleural cavity via medical thoracoscopy and try to resolve the pleuropulmonary adhesions.

Thoracic surgeon

It should be sufficient to exclude malignant pleural involvement. However, the visceral pleura looks quite thick on the CT scan; therefore I'm not sure if you can free the lung with thoracoscopy. With more time passing, the risk of decortication becomes greater.

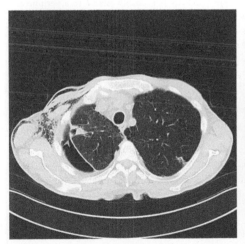 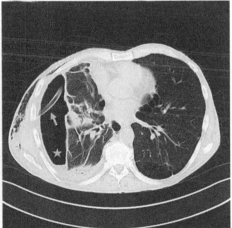

Fig. 11.4 Axial computed tomography (CT) scan, obtained 14 days after chest tube placement, showing an irregular subpleural lung hyperdensity, with internal cavitation and a thin communication with the pleural space in correspondence with the apical segment of the right upper lobe *(arrowhead)*. Pneumothorax is still present, with a small amount of fluid at the bottom of the pleural cavity *(star)*. The chest tube *(arrow)* and a small area of subcutaneous emphysema *(asterisk)* resulting from the procedure are also evident.

Bronchoscopy was performed and showed only a slight distortion and width reduction in the right principal bronchi, without evident endobronchial lesions or mucosal abnormalities.

The patient then underwent medical thoracoscopy, which revealed pleural thickening and tenacious adhesions mainly between the lung and the mediastinal pleura, and the operator could

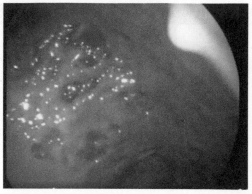

Fig. 11.5 Medical thoracoscopy view showing thickened parietal pleura with tenacious adhesions between the visceral and parietal pleurae.

not remove them (Fig. 11.5). Parietal pleural biopsies were performed, with the results of histology being negative for malignancy.

A chest tube was maintained for 8 more days, without any clinical or radiological improvement.

Discussion Topic

Thoracic surgeon

The persistence of air in the pleural cavity is probably related to a peripheral bronchopleural fistula. This is a serious complication, and its treatment is a challenge for thoracic surgeons.

Pneumologist B

Some bronchoscopic techniques, such as application of sealants, fibrin glue, coils, and endobronchial stents, have been proposed for the control of small bronchopleural fistulae (BPF).

Thoracic surgeon

There is no consensus on the most effective method for BPF closure. Endoscopic techniques are used only for patients in poor clinical condition. I suggest an appropriate major surgical intervention.

Pulmonologist A

Can we stop antibiotic therapy now?

Pulmonologist B

Yes, we can. Both cross-reactive protein (CRP) and procalcitonin (PCT) values are normal.

Discussion Topic—cont'd

Even the tube is no longer needed. No more air or liquid is coming out of the pleural cavity.

Thoracic surgeon

Subsequently, surgery was proposed. The patient underwent thoracotomy with lysis of adhesions, suture of the perforation at the upper right lobe that had caused the air leak, and decortication to allow lung re-expansion.

Radiological findings were significantly altered, and the right lung was expanded more (Fig. 11.6).

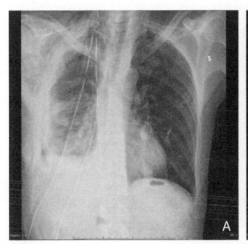
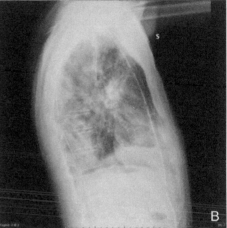

Fig. 11.6 Chest radiography (A: posteroanterior; B: lateral) obtained soon after surgery showing expanded right lung and chest tube placement.

Follow-Up and Outcomes

One month after discharge, the patient was afebrile and experienced breathlessness only during effort. After removal of the thoracic drainage, the right lung remained expanded, and no recurrences of pneumothorax were observed.

Focus On

Ultrasound Appearance of Empyema

Pleural empyema is defined as the presence of pus in the pleural cavity; the pus is a purulent exudate consisting of plasma with a high concentration of both active and dead leukocytes, predominantly neutrophils. On ultrasonography, this can appear as anechoic pleural fluid with hyperechoic debris within it. A similar appearance can be found when pleural effusion contains blood (hemothorax), chyle (chylothorax), cholesterol (pseudochylothorax), or proteinaceous debris in other diseases, such as malignancies. Moreover, purulent pleural effusion may become loculated with multiple fibrinous strands and adhesions.

Malignant pleural effusion should be considered in the differential diagnosis of loculated pleural effusions.

In the presence of pyopneumothorax, analysis of pus and air collected from the pleura and ultrasonography can reveal the presence of anechoic fluid containing multiple hyperechoic floating debris and microbubbles.

Focus On

Choice of the Chest Drain Insertion Site

Chest radiography and chest ultrasonography should always be performed before placing a chest tube, except in urgent situations, such as hypertensive pneumothorax. Images from chest computed tomography (CT) can provide additional information.

Imaging helps evaluate the characteristics of the pleural content and select the appropriate site for chest tube placement.

The most common site for chest tube insertion for pleural effusion is at or just above the fifth intercostal space on the midaxillary line, in the so-called "safe triangle." This is an area with thin muscle layers, delimited anteriorly by the lateral edge of the pectoralis major, posteriorly by the lateral edge of the latissimus dorsi, and inferiorly by the fifth intercostal space, usually identified at the level of the nipple.

The choice of this site minimizes the risk of damaging vital structures, such as the internal mammary artery; prevents cutting and passing of the tube through large muscles, such as the pectoralis major and breast tissue; and avoids unsightly scarring. Moreover, the safe triangle is usually causes the least discomfort for the patient.

A more posterior position is also safe, but the patient cannot lie on the back, and the tube has a higher risk of kinking or dislocating.

In the case of loculated pleural effusion, the drain must be inserted in the chest wall area corresponding to the pleural effusion, and ultrasound guidance is essential to identify that area.

It is common to insert the chest tube by using the so-called free-hand technique, in which the physician marks the entry point under ultrasound guidance and perform the procedure immediately afterward while the patient stays still.

The insertion site for apical pneumothorax or hypertensive pneumothorax is often the second intercostal space on the hemiclavicular line. However, this is not recommended routinely because it may cause discomfort for the patient and an unsightly scar.

Particular cases, such as loculated pneumothorax, require placement of the chest tube in the affected area. For instance, loculated apical pneumothorax, which can rarely occur after thoracotomy, may be drained by using a posterior suprascapular chest tube placed by an operator experienced in this technique.

Before insertion, air or fluid should be aspirated with a needle at the time of anaesthesia to confirm the right position.

Once the intercostal space has been chosen, the thoracic tube must be positioned along the upper edge of the lower rib, to avoid the neurovascular bundle.

The direction of the insertion of the tube depends on the pathology being treated. The tube should be directed anteriorly and toward the apex to drain pneumothorax or posteriorly to drain pleural effusion.

Focus On

Bronchopleural Fistula

Bronchopleural fistula (BPF) is a pathological communication between the bronchial tree and the pleural space. It is a potential complication that occurs after pneumonectomy or other pulmonary resection, but other causes, including necrotizing pneumonia, lung neoplasm, persistent spontaneous pneumothorax, blunt or penetrating lung injuries, and tuberculosis, have also been documented.

Management of BPF requires prolonged hospitalization, complex surgical procedures, and close follow-up. A chest tube must be applied as soon as possible to ensure drainage of the pleural cavity. Broad-spectrum antibiotic therapy against gram-positive, gram-negative, and anaerobic microorganisms must be initiated, but it should be tailored on the basis of the results of culture antibiograms.

Treatment for BPF ranges from medical management to bronchoscopic procedures in critically ill patients and surgical intervention in those deemed to be at the highest risk.

So far, there is lack of consensus regarding the optimal management of BPF because of varying reports of therapeutic success.

LEARNING POINTS

- Chest ultrasonography can stratify parapneumonic pleural effusion in free-flowing and multiloculated pleural empyema, thus helping diagnosis and guiding therapeutic interventions.
- Complicated parapneumonic pleural effusion and empyema require quick treatment through chest tube placement or more invasive procedures.
- Trapped lung may require medical thoracoscopy, video-assisted thoracoscopic surgery (VATS) or open surgical decortication.
- Necrotizing pneumonia can be complicated by an alveolar–pleural or bronchopleural fistula, resulting in pyopneumothorax.

Further Reading

1. Davies HE, Davies RJO, Davies CWH. on behalf of the BTS Pleural Disease Guideline Group. Management of pleural infection in adults: British Thoracic Society pleural disease guideline 2010. *Thorax.* 2010;65(Suppl 2):ii41–ii53.
2. Brutsche MH, Tassi G, Györik S, et al. Treatment of sonographically stratified multiloculated thoracic empyema by medical thoracoscopy. *Chest.* 2005;128:3303–3309.
3. Sarkar P, Chandak T, Shah R, Talwar A. Diagnosis and management bronchopleural Fistula. *Indian J Chest Dis Allied Sci.* 2010;52(2):97–104.
4. Chalmers JD, Singanayagam A, Murray MP, Scally C, Fawzi A, Hill AT. Risk factors for complicated parapneumonic effusion and empyema on presentation to hospital with community-acquired pneumonia. *Thorax.* 2009;64(7):592–597.
5. Huggins JT, Maldonado F, Chopra A, et al. Unexpandable lung from pleural disease. *Respirology.* 2018;23(2):160–167.

CHAPTER 12

Pneumonia and Volume Overload Complicating Chronic Fibrothorax With Persistent Fluid Collection

Stefano Elia ■ Claudio Sorino ■ Giampietro Marchetti ■ Stefano Negri ■ Natalia Buda

History of Present Illness

An 83-year-old man was taken to the emergency room (ER) because of fever, shortness of breath, swelling of the legs, weakness, confusion, and nausea.

Past Medical History

The patient suffered from arterial hypertension, hyperuricemia, type 2 diabetes mellitus, diabetic nephropathy with proteinuria, and stage 4 chronic kidney disease. An indwelling peritoneal catheter had recently been implanted because peritoneal dialysis was considered a therapeutic option (not yet started). Many years earlier, the patient had been diagnosed with left fibrothorax with fluid collection resulting from previous tuberculous pleurisy.

Physical Examination and Early Clinical Findings

Upon arrival at the ER, the patient had a fever (38.7° C [101.7° F]) and low oxygen saturation (oxygen saturation [SpO_2] 87% at rest while breathing in ambient air). Arterial blood gas (ABG) analyses showed metabolic acidosis and acute partial respiratory failure (pH 7.28; partial pressure of carbon dioxide [$PaCO_2$] 39.3 mm Hg; partial pressure of oxygen [PaO_2] 54.8 mm Hg; bicarbonate [HCO_3-] 14 mmol/L). Respiratory rate was 21 breaths/min, heart rate was 114 beats/min, and arterial blood pressure was 130/85 mm Hg. Auscultation revealed a reduction in vesicular murmur in the left lower field, crackles in the right middle and basal fields, and widespread rales. Chest x-ray showed large opacity in the left middle and lower areas and opacity in the right middle zone (Fig. 12.1). Chest ultrasonography confirmed the presence of fluid collection and calcified pleura on the left side. Moreover, lung hepatization with air bronchogram in the left lower lobe was seen (Fig. 12.2).

Blood tests showed leukocytosis (white blood cells [WBC] count: 18,200/mm³) and a marked increase in the indices of inflammation (C-reactive protein [CRP]: 330 mg/L; procalcitonin [PCT]: 1.56 mcg/L) and volume overload (N-terminal–pro–brain natriuretic peptide [NT-proBNP]: 13,650 pg/mL). Renal failure, hyperglycemia, and electrolyte imbalance were also evident: serum creatinine was 5.3 mg/dL, glucose 215 mg/dL, and potassium 5.8 mEq/L. Urinalysis revealed the presence of leukocytes, hemoglobin, proteins, glucose, and bacteria in urine.

Supplemental 40% oxygen via a Venturi mask was delivered to obtain oxygen saturation of 96%. A loop diuretic (intravenous furosemide, bolus dose of 40 mg, followed by continuous infusion of 0.1 mg/kg/h) and a broad-spectrum antibiotic with dose adjustment for renal impairment (intravenous meropenem 500 mg every 24 hours) were promptly initiated. The patient was admitted to the nephrology unit.

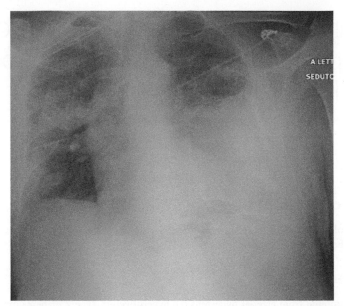

Fig. 12.1 A chest radiograph showing large opacity in the left middle and lower areas, suggesting pleural thickening and calcification. Opacity in the right middle zone is also evident.

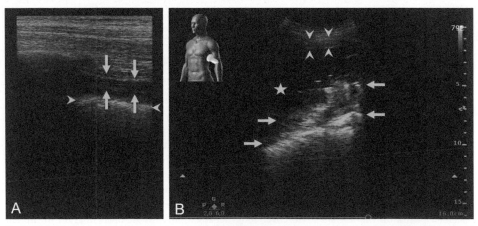

Fig. 12.2 Left chest ultrasonography image. (A) Linear probe: thickness of parietal pleura *(vertical arrows)* and pleural line *(arrowheads)*. (B) Convex probe: hepatization of the lung with air bronchogram in left lower lobe *(horizontal arrows),* pleural effusion *(star),* and thickened parietal pleura *(arrowheads).*

Discussion Topic

Nephrologist

The chest radiograph is not of excellent quality. Radiography was performed bedside, with the patient supine, in a single anteroposterior projection.

Discussion Topic—cont'd

Pulmonologist A

I agree. The large left opacity is difficult to interpret. We know that the patient has fibrothorax there. However, it can mask an infection, a tumor, or pleural effusion. Instead the right hemithorax opacity could be pneumonia.

Pulmonologist B

Could chest ultrasonography help understand the left findings?

Pulmonologist A

Probably yes. However, the calcifications of fibrothorax are a bad acoustic window. I'm not sure if we can properly evaluate the lung and the pleural cavity. Surely CT will have to be performed.

Nephrologist

What do you think about the vertical line on the right hemithorax? Could it be pneumothorax?

Pulmonologist A

Absolutely not. In the case of pneumothorax, we would see homogeneous external radiolucency. Here, however, the pulmonary pattern is well recognizable. These images are frequently produced on radiographs performed on a supine or seated patient because of the skin folds produced by contact of the patient's back with a hard surface.

Nephrologist

The patient may have a reactivation of tuberculosis (TB). Would the QuantiFERON TB test or the tuberculin skin test be useful?

Pulmonologist B

These tests only have a role in identifying latent TB. However, we already know that the patient had TB! To diagnose active TB, we must search for tuberculous bacilli or their genetic material in suitable samples.

Nephrologist

Would you try thoracentesis?

Pulmonologist A

It wouldn't be easy because of calcified fibrothorax. I would avoid it and start with sputum smear microscopy and culture. Let's see the clinical evolution and discuss it again after chest CT.

Clinical Course

The day after admission, serum creatinine increased to 6.8 mg/dL. Urine output was low (about 100 mL/24 hr). The physicians proposed hemodialysis, but the patient refused it; thus peritoneal dialysis was started. Kayexalate, oral sodium bicarbonate, and insulin, in addition to antibiotics and a diuretic, were administered. Glycated hemoglobin (HbA1c), measured to determine the 3-month average blood glucose level, was high (8.1%) and confirmed uncontrolled diabetes. Sputum smear microscopy was negative for acid-fast bacilli (AFB), as well as the search for *Mycobacterium tuberculosis* DNA by means of polymerase chain reaction (PCR) on three consecutive sputum samples. The urine culture was positive for *Proteus mirabilis*, but no aerobic or anaerobic microorganism growth was detected on blood cultures. In 3 days, the fever disappeared, and the patient experienced progressive clinical improvement.

Discussion Topic

Nephrologist

The patient is much better. Sputum microbiological tests all showed negative results. Do you still think he may have active tuberculosis (TB)?

Pulmonologist A

If yes, we should treat it. In case of uncertainty, we could give ex juvantibus therapy to prevent TB spread.

Pulmonologist B

I would not initiate anti-TB therapy without evidence of active TB and results from drug susceptibility tests. The patient was previously treated for this and should take at least three medications for several months. They can have considerable side effects.

Pulmonologist A

I wouldn't be satisfied with negative results from smear and culture on sputum. I think we should perform bronchoscopy with mycobacterial analysis of bronchoalveolar lavage (BAL) fluid.

Nephrologist

I'd wait to see the CT scan. This hasn't been performed yet.

Pulmonologist A

Ok, but I'd perform bronchoscopy anyway. If this also shows negative results, we can reasonably rule out active pulmonary TB.

Pulmonologist B

And what if the bacilli were in the pleural cavity? Antibiotics wouldn't get there.

Discussion Topic—cont'd

Pulmonologist A

Sorry to ask again: could you try to aspirate the fluid inside the fibrothorax?

Pulmonologist C

In my opinion, it isn't a good idea. Touching the tuberculous sequelae is not recommended, especially when they are calcified, unless the patient has persistent symptoms and signs of inflammation.

Chest computed tomography (CT) was not feasible for a few days because of technical problems. The patient underwent bronchoscopy, which showed a diffusely atrophic and inflamed bronchial mucosa. Some mucous secretions from both bronchial hemisystems were aspirated, and bronchoalveolar lavage (BAL) was performed in the lower left lobe. The recovered BAL fluid was analyzed, and no mycobacteria or malignant tumor cells were found.

In a week, edema in the lower limbs decreased, and oxygen saturation became sufficient without administration of oxygen. The WBC count normalized, and the CRP value decreased to 28 mg/L.

Chest radiography and CT showed that the pulmonary opacities in the middle right and lower left areas had disappeared. The pulmonary opacity caused by the known left calcific fibrothorax was still very evident (Figs. 12.3 and 12.4).

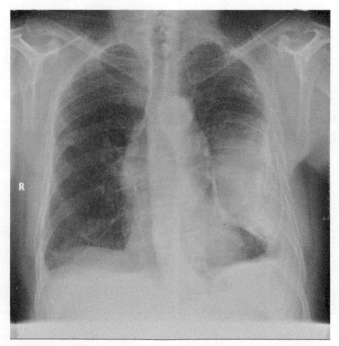

Fig. 12.3 Chest radiograph obtained after resolution of pneumonia, clearly showing the shape of fibrothorax. The convex medial margin clearly indicates the presence of liquid between the visceral pleura and the parietal pleura. Fibrothoraces with liquid content produce high-density peripheral lines on the chest radiograph, corresponding to the pleural sections that are reached tangentially by the x-rays.

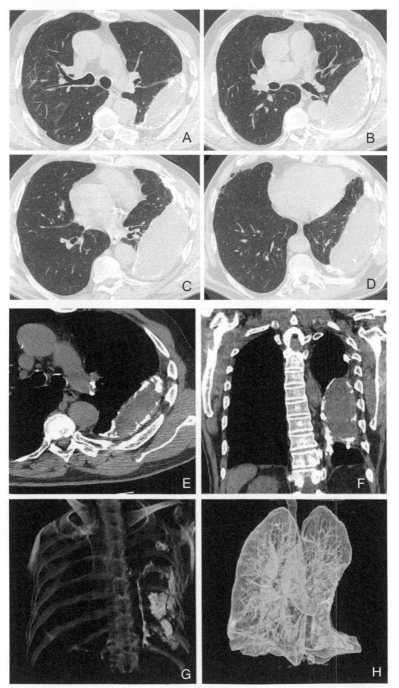

Fig. 12.4 Chest computed tomography (CT) scan after pneumonia resolution. (A–D) Parenchymal window showing absence of lung lesions, except for the left fibrothorax area. The fibrothorax with fluid content is clearly evident in the mediastinal window (E and F, respectively, in the axial and coronal planes). The three-dimensional reconstruction (G) shows discontinuously calcified walls of the fibrothorax. The volume rendering (H) clearly define the extension of the fibrothorax and its effects on lung expansion.

Antibiotic therapy was continued until the CRP level dropped to normal values (for a total of 12 days), and intravenous furosemide was converted to an appropriate oral dose.

Recommended Therapy and Further Indications at Discharge

In consideration of the positive outcome, the patient was discharged home with instructions to continue the peritoneal dialysis and to ensure clinical and radiological follow-up of the pulmonary lesion. He was instructed to continue long-acting insulin therapy (insulin glargine, 14 units at bedtime) plus a rapid-acting insulin analogue (insulin glulisine, 5–10 units before meals, according to preprandial capillary blood glucose). Because of residual renal function (urine volume about 200 mL/day), the patient was kept on oral furosemide 500 mg once daily.

Follow-Up and Outcomes

In the month after discharge, the patient did not have any fever or respiratory symptoms, except for mild exertional dyspnea. The same condition had existed before the event that caused hospitalization. Chest radiography showed unchanged findings. Upon an outpatient visit to the pneumology department, spirometry was performed, and it showed a mild restrictive ventilatory defect. No respiratory therapy was prescribed.

Focus On

Definition, Causes, and Mechanism of Fibrothorax

Fibrothorax is the accumulation of dense fibrous tissue in the pleural cavity, also called *diffuse pleural thickening* or *pleural peel*.

The definition of fibrothorax is somewhat arbitrary. Many agree on a diagnosis of fibrothorax when the thickening of pleura is greater than 5 mm and extends continuously for 8 cm vertically and 5 cm laterally. According to others, pleural thickening that involves greater than 25% of the chest wall, if bilateral, and 50%, if unilateral, is to be considered fibrothorax.

Fibrothorax is caused by an intense inflammatory response, usually as a consequence of undrained complicated pleural effusion. This results in the deposition of fibrin between the pleural surfaces and sometimes in the fusion of visceral and parietal pleura into a single layer of fibrous tissue, which often becomes calcified. Fibrothorax can affect one or both hemithoraces and may have persistent or recurrent fluid collection inside it. As a consequence, lung expansion becomes difficult, and atelectasis may occur. Hemithorax is contracted, intercostal spaces are narrowed, and the mediastinum is attracted. The reduced lung volumes determine a restrictive ventilatory pattern. The most frequent causes of fibrothorax are hemothorax, tuberculous pleurisy, and complicated parapneumonic effusion/empyema. It can also develop as a result of asbestos exposure, collagen vascular disease, and drug-induced pleuritis (e.g., ergot derivatives), therapeutic pneumothorax, and pleurodesis. In most cases, ribs and intercostal muscles are intact and allow lung re-expansion after decortication. However, occasionally fibrosis can involve the intercostal muscles, incorporate the endothoracic fascia, and merge with the periosteum of the ribs.

Focus On

Imaging of Fibrothorax

Fibrothorax is often recognizable on plain chest radiographs. One of the most common features is the extensive and gross thickening of the pleura. It is mainly, but not exclusively, one-sided, and spares the interlobar fissures. Pleural thickening is generally continuous, smooth, and regular, without nodulations, and has a variable extension from the bases upward. Viewed in profile, it appears as a band of soft tissue density almost parallel to the chest wall. Viewed frontally, it appears as ill-defined, veil-like shadowing.

Continued

Focus On—cont'd

It can be associated with reduction in the intercostal spaces and the size of the involved hemithorax, with consequent ipsilateral attraction of the mediastinum and a hemidiaphragm rise.

Pleural thickening may involve the parietal and visceral pleurae, which are often blended together. Thickness can range from 2 to 10 mm (up to 20 mm if the sum of parietal and visceral pleurae is considered). Therefore a thickening greater than 20 mm, as seen on the chest radiograph, associated with the typical characteristics of fibrothorax cannot be explained only by the presence of fibrotic tissue, and the coexistence of pleural effusion should be investigated.

It can affect the diaphragm, the costodiaphragmatic recesses, and the chest wall, whereas the mediastinal pleura is not commonly affected. If thickening involves mediastinal pleura, mesothelioma or other malignancies should be suspected.

Pleural calcifications that appear as "cuttlefish bone" can also be found and are quite extensive in patients with previous tuberculosis infection.

Chest ultrasonography allows for rapid bedside evaluation of the patient and may help in the differential diagnosis. Fibrothorax is usually detectable on ultrasonography if the thickness is greater than 10 mm. It appears as a homogeneous echogenic layer inside the chest wall, covering the lung. The pleural line is thickened, and the "gliding sign" is attenuated.

Chest computed tomography (CT) (better if high-resolution CT) is also useful for diagnosis. It allows for accurate recognition of pleural thickening and for distinguishing it from extrapleural fat (between the pleura and the intercostal muscle or the rib). Moreover, CT may identify coexisting interstitial lung fibrosis caused by asbestos exposure and quantify lung damage extension, which aids in risk/benefit evaluation in candidates for pleurectomy.

Focus On

Fibrothorax and Decortication of the Lung

Decortication of the lung is a surgical procedure involving removal of the thick, inelastic layer of fibrous tissue surrounding an entrapped lung, to allow its re-expansion.

In many cases, the fibrous peel may spontaneously resolve. Early pharmacological treatment and minor interventions, including chest tube placement, irrigation, and thoracoscopic debridement, can help avoid major surgery. Despite such procedures, organization and entrapment of the lung may still occur, and decortication remains the treatment of choice. The main indications for decortication are the presence of fibrothorax for longer than 4 to 6 weeks, disabling respiratory symptoms, and radiological evidence of trapped lung. Patient selection is important because decortication can be a very bloody procedure. Timing of surgery is equally important because decortication gives the best results in patients who seek early treatment. If the disease has been chronic, several technical problems arise, both with regard to entry into the thorax (the spaces of the ribs are often melted, the thoracic cavity is severely restricted) and removal of the peel (which becomes thick up to a few centimeters, and adherent to the lung).

Relative contraindications for decortication are uncontrolled lung infections or severe chest wall infections, contralateral lung diseases, coagulopathy, terminal diseases, or the presence of chronic debilitation. An underlying lung disease, pleural space infection, and large-airway stenosis are conditions that may prevent lung re-expansion despite decortication. The patient should be carefully assessed for these conditions to avoid futile surgery.

Bronchoscopy should be performed before decortication to identify any large-airway pathology (e.g., bronchial stenosis, malignancy) that may be the cause of lung collapse.

For a long time, decortication was performed only through thoracotomy. Today, video-assisted thoracoscopic surgery (VATS) is a valid alternative that has been associated with better outcomes, less pain, and faster recovery compared with the open approach.

During the procedure, the patient is intubated, and the surgery is done with the patient under general anesthesia. Single-lung ventilation is rarely necessary because the trapped lung is usually already compressed as a result of the fibrothorax. The goal is to remove all the fibrinous layers and necrotic tissue to promote lung re-expansion.

The two main problems in performing decortication are pleural cavity infection and fibrosis.

Pleuropulmonary complications associated with decortication are infections, bronchopleural fistulas, bleeding, and persistent air leakage (most air leaks seal within a few days, but large leaks may persist for weeks). Patients with borderline lung function are more likely to develop respiratory distress in the postoperative period compared with those with better lung function.

LEARNING POINTS

- Fibrothorax is diffuse pleural thickening and occasionally has fluid collection inside.
- Early drainage and/or debridement of complicated pleural effusion can prevent fibrothorax.
- Fibrothorax is a relevant cause of restrictive ventilatory defects.
- Decortication may allow lung re-expansion in patients with chronic fibrothorax and lung entrapment.
- Pre-existing fibrothorax may confound imaging findings of pneumonia.

Further Reading

1. Jants MA, Antony VB. Pleural fibrosis. *Clin Chest Med.* 2006;27(2):181–191.
2. Asri H, Zegmout A. Historic sequelae of lung tuberculosis. *Pan Afr Med J.* 2018;30:210.
3. Irfan M. Post-tuberculosis pulmonary function and noninfectious pulmonary disorders. *Int J Mycobacteriol.* 2016;5(Suppl 1):S57.
4. Donath J, Miller A. Restrictive chest wall disorders. *Semin Respir Crit Care Med.* 2009;30(3):275–292.
5. Schmitt WGH, Hubener KH, Rucker HC. Pleural calcification with persistent effusion. *Radiology.* 1983;149(3):633–638.
6. Nichkaode PB, Agrawal R, Patel SK. Thoracotomy and decortication in chronic empyema (fibrothorax) in the era of video assisted thoracic surgery. *Int Surg J.* 2017;4(8):2741–2745.
7. Cohen AM, Crass JR, Chung-Park M, Tomashefski Jr JF. Rounded atelectasis and fibrotic pleural disease: the pathologic continuum. *J Thorac Imaging.* 1993;8(4):309–312.
8. Gorman J, Funk D, Srinathan S, et al. Perioperative implications of thoracic decortications: a retrospective cohort study. *Can J Anaesth.* 2017;64(8):845–853.

CHAPTER 13

Late Postpneumonectomy Bronchopleural Fistula With Pleural Empyema

Fabrizio Minervini ▦ Marco Scarci ▦ Claudio Sorino ▦ Pietro Bertoglio

History of Present Illness

A 62-year-old Caucasian female patient presented to the emergency room with new-onset sputum production, fatigue, and fever. Chest radiography showed air–fluid level in the left thoracic cavity (Fig. 13.1).

Past Medical History

The patient was a former smoker (20 cigarettes a day; 35 pack-years). She stopped smoking 8 years before the current episode, when she had been diagnosed with non–small cell lung cancer and underwent left upper lobectomy with mediastinal radical lymphadenectomy. Seven years after that surgery, the patient had undergone left completion pneumonectomy for hemoptysis caused by aspergilloma. Chronic obstructive pulmonary disease (COPD) had been also diagnosed, with moderate airway obstruction, and a long-acting muscarinic agent (tiotropium Respimat 2.5 µg, two inhalations in the morning) was ordered. However, the patient did not take it regularly.

Physical Examination and Early Clinical Findings

Upon arrival at the hospital, the patient was alert and oriented but appeared cachectic, pale, and fatigued. She was febrile (body temperature 38.1° C [100.58° F]) and had a blood pressure of 96/62 mm Hg, heart rate of 107 beats/min, respiratory rate of 25 breaths/min, and oxygen saturation of 86% at pulse oximeter. Arterial blood gas (ABG) analysis in room air showed normal pH (7.39), hypoxemia (partial pressure of oxygen [PaO_2] 55.4 mm Hg), slight hypercapnia (partial pressure of carbon dioxide [$PaCO_2$] 47.2 mm Hg), and rise of bicarbonate (HCO_3^- 28 mEq/L). Respiratory examination revealed absence of breath sounds on the left side of the chest and no pathological findings on the right side. Cardiovascular examination was unremarkable. The abdomen was soft, without distension or ascites.

Diagnostic laboratory workup for infection showed a marked elevation of inflammatory parameters (serum C-reactive protein [CRP] 296 mg/L; normal values < 5 mg/L) and leukocytosis (white blood cell [WBC] count 10,700 cells/µL, neutrophils 87%). Lactate was slightly increased (2 mmol/L).

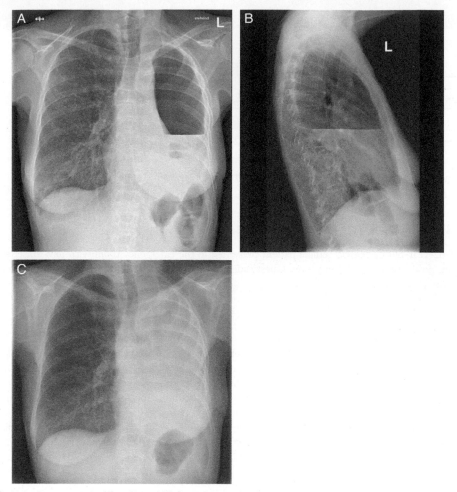

Fig. 13.1 Posteroanterior (A) and lateral (B) chest radiographs showing a large air–fluid level in the left hemithorax. A previous posteroanterior chest radiograph (C) showed complete fluid filling of the postpneumonectomy space.

Discussion Topic

ER doctor

I just visited the patient with previous pneumonectomy. Now she has hypercapnic respiratory failure and probably a pleural cavity infection.

Pulmonologist A

I saw her arterial blood gas (ABG) results: Blood pH is normal, and bicarbonate increased. It is very likely that the patient has chronic carbon dioxide (CO_2) retention. I recommend giving supplemental oxygen at the minimum level necessary to obtain oxygen saturation (SpO_2) greater than 90% or partial pressure of oxygen (PaO_2) greater than 60 mm Hg.

So we will reduce the risk of central respiratory depression, which would cause hypoventilation and further increase in $PaCO_2$.

Discussion Topic—cont'd

ER doctor

One year after pneumonectomy, the chest cavity should be filled with fluid. I would have expected complete opacification of the hemithorax.

Pulmonologist A

I fear the patient has a bronchopleural fistula (BPF). We should refer her to a thoracic surgeon.

ER doctor

Do you think that thoracic drainage would be useful? We could analyze the pleural fluid and obtain cultures.

Pulmonologist A

I believe that a conservative approach is not an option. The patient probably needs surgery right away!

ER doctor

I ordered intravenous fluids to reduce the risk of blood pressure going dangerously low. We also need to initiate antibiotic therapy. What do you advise?

Pulmonologist A

If a BPF is present, we should use broad-spectrum intravenous agents against gram-positive, gram-negative, and anaerobic microorganisms. I suggest a combination regimen with piperacillin/tazobactam, vancomycin, and levofloxacin, which can also protect against methicillin-resistant *Staphylococcus aureus* (MRSA) and *Pseudomonas aeruginosa*.

We should also optimize therapy for comorbidities—in particular, reintroduce bronchodilators—and ensure adequate nutrition.

Clinical Course

The patient initially received 50% oxygen supplement via a Venturi mask and obtained oxygen saturation (SpO_2) of 98%. According to the pulmonologist's recommendation, supplemental oxygen was reduced to 3 L/min administered via a nasal cannula, and SpO_2 of 92% to 94% was maintained.

Intravenous fluid therapy with a crystalloid solution (Ringer's lactate solution [RLS] 60 mL/hr) was initiated, in addition to intravenous antibiotics (piperacillin/tazobactam 4.5 g every 8 hours, vancomycin 500 mg every 6 hours, and levofloxacin 750 mg once a day). Blood cultures were obtained before antibiotics were administered. A urinary catheter was placed to monitor urine output. After checking for hemodynamic stability, the patient was admitted to the thoracic surgery unit.

Discussion Topic

Thoracic surgeon A

Chest radiography has shown a significant reduction in pleural fluid in the chest cavity. Moreover, the increased air content causes a slight contralateral shift of the mediastinum. I agree with your hypothesis. These findings, the medical history, and the symptoms all point to a bronchopleural fistula (BPF)!

Pulmonologist B

It's been a long time since the surgery. What usually happens in the chest cavity after the lung is removed?

Thoracic surgeon B

Immediately after pneumonectomy, air fills the space previously occupied by the lung. Over time, a number of changes result in a decrease in the size of the postpneumonectomy space. Usually the hemidiaphragm elevates, the remaining lung hyperinflates, and the mediastinum shifts toward the empty hemithorax. At the same time, air is progressively reabsorbed and replaced by fluid.

Thoracic surgeon A

This usually occurs in 1 month to 7 months. If a patient still has an air–fluid level in the chest cavity and if it drops by 2 cm or greater, it is likely that a BPF has occurred.

Pulmonologist B

However, chest radiography may indicate a BPF. I think bronchoscopy is important to confirm it on the basis of direct or indirect signs and to assess its extent.

Pulmonologist A

Bronchial endoscopy may show false-negative results, especially in the case of small-sized fistulas. You can do an endoscopic evaluation, but I believe that chest radiography would clearly indicate the diagnosis of BPF.

Pulmonologist B

In case of doubt, methylene blue can be released into the bronchi, and then its presence in the chest drain can be verified.

Thoracic surgeon A

Chest computed tomography (CT) is also indicated. Multidetector CT has good sensitivity, similar to bronchoscopy.

Pulmonologist B

Virtual bronchoscopy and ventilation scintigraphy have been also described in the diagnostic path for bronchopleural fistula (BPF). However, we need a quick diagnosis because further surgical treatment may be indicated.

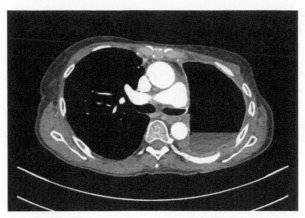

Fig. 13.2 Computed tomography (CT) scan showing air–fluid level, enhancement of the parietal pleura, and air near the left bronchial stump.

The suspicion of a fistula between the left bronchial stump and the pneumonectomy space was confirmed with chest computed tomography (CT) (Fig. 13.2) and bronchoscopy (Fig. 13.3).

Posterolateral thoracotomy was performed the day after admission, and loculated, smelly pleural effusion was found intraoperatively. After extensive debridement of the necrotic and fibrous infected tissue, the left thoracic cavity was irrigated with saline. Because of the short stump, a direct closure or shortening of the left main bronchus was not possible. Thus the thoracic surgeons decided to use the omentum as a patch. Short upper laparotomy was performed, and the omentum was dissected from the stomach along the greater curvature and released from the transverse colon and mesocolon. Through a small incision of the diaphragm, the omentum was placed in the left thoracic cavity. It was then sutured on the bronchial wall with five interrupted sutures. To ensure a tension-free flap, the omentum was fixed to the mediastinal pleura. At the end of the procedure, the surgeons packed the left thoracic cavity with four gauzes impregnated with povidone-iodine solution. Then a chest tube was inserted and the thoracotomy temporarily closed. Continuous

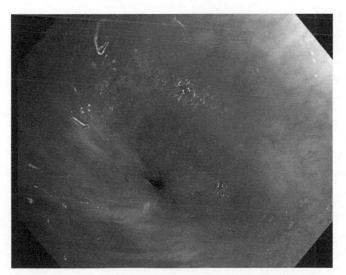

Fig. 13.3 Bronchoscopic view of the bronchopleural fistula (BPF). A mucosal defect was present at the surgical site (left main bronchial stump), with bubbling of saline when instilled.

suction of 5 mm Hg was applied through the chest tube. The patient was extubated in the operating room and transferred to the intermediate care unit. The antiseptic packing was changed on the second and fourth postoperative days. On postoperative day 6, the operative field was macroscopically clean; therefore the clinicians decided to fill the cavity with 1 L of saline, which also contained 0.3 of netilmicin, 2.2 g of amoxicillin/clavulanic acid, 1 g of vancomycin, and 0.4 g of fluconazole. The patient was discharged from the hospital 15 days after surgery.

Discussion Topic

Pulmonologist A

The treatment of choice of bronchopleural fistula (BPF) is surgery, isn't it?

Thoracic surgeon A

Management of a BPF strictly depends on its size, the time of its appearance (early or late), and the clinical condition of the patient. In case of an early-stage BPF, surgical repair is usually the preferred treatment, whereas a late-stage fistula is usually treated with open-window thoracostomy, followed by delayed surgical repair.

Thoracic surgeon B

Nevertheless, in patients who are not fit for surgery, conservative approaches should be offered. Chest cavity drainage is always mandatory. Different kinds of bio-glues, coils, or silver nitrate can be used to try to close the fistula endoscopically.

Thoracic surgeon A

A similar choice can also be made in the case of a small-sized fistula, usually less than 8 mm in size.

Pulmonologist B

Is there any role for airway stenting?

Pulmonologist A

Stenting of the airway with the aim of sealing and isolating the fistula has been proposed and described in case reports. However, both Dumont stents and covered metallic stents have shown inconsistent results.

Recommended Therapy and Further Indications at Discharge

Chest radiography performed 7 days after surgery showed almost complete filling of the postpneumonectomy cavity with fluid. Intravenous antibiotic therapy was continued for a total of 15 days, after which the patient was discharged with instructions to take oral amoxicillin/clavulanic acid 875/125 mg every 8 hours for another 10 days.

Inhaled therapy with tiotropium Respimat was administrated throughout hospitalization because use of this device did not require inhalation effort. The physicians stressed the importance of adherence to inhalation therapy at home. The patient also received high-calorie food supplements to improve her nutritional status.

Follow-Up and Outcomes

The patient followed up in the outpatient clinic 6 weeks and 12 weeks after surgery. Chest radiography showed complete opacification of the left hemithorax, without presence of air. The patient remained afebrile and experienced episodes of mild chest pain, which were well controlled by paracetamol as needed.

Focus On

Strategies to Prevent Postpneumonectomy Empyema

Postpneumonectomy empyema is a life-threatening complication of pneumonectomy. It is often related to the development of a bronchopleural fistula (BPF), which allows airway bacteria to colonize the chest cavity.

The most well-known risk factors for the development of BFS and postpneumonectomy empyema are right-side pneumonectomy, surgery for benign disease, poor pulmonary function, and low preoperative albumin levels. Moreover, neoadjuvant therapies, diabetes, chronic use of steroids or immunosuppressive drugs, and age have also been reported as potential risk factors.

Technical aspects that might reduce the incidence of BPF are of paramount importance. In particular, thoracic surgeons should reduce the length of the bronchial stump to a minimum and preserve bronchial vascularization as much as possible. Moreover, to obtain cancer-free bronchial margins, it is important to both ensure a radical resection and prevent the development of BPF. However, data on the closure technique (either mechanical or manual) of the bronchial stump are inconsistent, and no conclusions can be drawn. Last, coverage of bronchial stump with healthy viable tissue seems to be an advisable procedure because it carries a very low risk of complication; thus it is routinely used in high-risk patients.

Concurrent anesthetic management is also important. Prolonged intubation with mechanical ventilation causes persistent barotrauma on the bronchial suture; it has been recognized as an independent risk factor for the development of BPF and thus should be avoided.

Focus On

Management of Postpneumonectomy Empyema

The management of postpneumonectomy empyema represents a challenge for thoracic surgeons, and to date there is no consensus regarding the best treatment for it. Several surgical approaches have been proposed, but their use depends on the individual surgeon's preference and experience. Open-window thoracostomy (Clagett's procedure) is a three-stage procedure first described in 1963 by Dr. Oscar Clagett and is still being used in the management of postpneumonectomy empyema. The removal of two or three ribs is done to leave an opening in the chest wall, allowing for repeated drainage, irrigation, and dressing of the cavity. It may represent a definitive solution while waiting for the gradual tissue granulation of the thoracic cavity until closure over time, or it can also be a bridge to secondary wound closure through a muscle or an omental flap once the infection of the pleural cavity has been healed. Modified Clagett's window was proposed by Pairolero et al. from the Mayo Clinic. In addition to the original procedure, they reinforced the bronchopleural fistula (BPF) with transposition of muscles (serratus anterior, latissimus dorsi, pectoralis major, pectoralis minor, or rectus abdominis). After observation of a clean pleural cavity, the space is obliterated with antibiotic solution and then closed.

Several years later, in 2001, Schneiter et al. described the surgical approach reported in the present case (i.e., an accelerated therapy with closure of the BPF and reinforcement with either a muscle flap or the omentum). These authors obtained definitive closure of chest within 8 days in 94.6% of patients and a low mortality rate of 4% at 90 days. The consequent disadvantages were the necessity for two or more additional surgeries and a prolonged length of hospital stay.

To achieve more efficient induction of tissue granulation and space obliteration, Perentes et al. proposed a treatment based on the procedure initially described by Pairolero but with the additional use of negative pressure wound therapy application by using a vacuum-assisted closure (VAC) device.

Focus On

Minimally Invasive Surgery for Postpneumonectomy Empyema

Minimally invasive surgery is currently gaining popularity as a fundamental approach in the field of thoracic surgery, and it might be safely used in complex cases by experts. Randomized controlled trials have demonstrated its benefit in terms of postoperative pain and length of hospital stay, and it has become the current standard of care in the majority of patients requiring lung resections.

Management of postpneumonectomy empyema with the use of video-assisted thoracoscopic surgery (VATS) has been reported in patients with postpneumonectomy empyema and no bronchopleural fistula (BPF) and in patients with postpneumonectomy empyema associated with a small-sized BPF (< 3 mm). In this selected subset of patients, an initial approach that is less aggressive than open-window thoracostomy may be reasonable and successful; VATS allows for effective debridement of the chest cavity (even though it offers an insufficient view of the costodiaphragmatic recess) and insertion of proper drainage that could be used for subsequent irrigation. Moreover, if necessary, VATS incisions allow for easy conversion to open-window thoracostomy. Results of observational cohort studies published in the literature have demonstrated the feasibility and safety of a minimally invasive approach in selected patients with postpneumonectomy empyema even with limited BPF. One of these studies reported the use of repeat VATS for chest cavity debridement of postpneumonectomy empyema. Furthermore, single case reports have also described the use of VATS for fistula suture and muscular flap transposition. In expert hands, VATS can play a role in the management of PPE.

LEARNING POINTS

- Prompt diagnosis of postpneumonectomy empyema and early treatment are essential to improve outcomes.
- Surgical and anesthetic strategies should be optimized to prevent postpneumonectomy empyema.
- In patients who are not fit for surgery or in cases of small-sized (< 8 mm) fistulas, a conservative approach may be offered, but in the majority of cases, surgery is the treatment of choice.

Further Reading

1. Clagett OT, Geraci JE. A procedure for the management of postpneumonectomy empyema. *J Thorac Cardiovasc Surg.* 1963;45:141–145.
2. Schneiter D, Cassina P, Korom S, et al. Accelerated treatment for early and late postpneumonectomy empyema. *Ann Thorac Surg.* 2001;72(5):1668–1672.
3. Schneiter D, Grodzki T, Lardinois D, et al. Accelerated treatment of postpneumonectomy empyema: a binational long-term study. *J Thorac Cardiovasc Surg.* 2008;136(1):179–185.
4. Liberman M, Cassivi SD. Bronchial stump dehiscence: update on prevention and management. *Semin Thorac Cardiovasc Surg.* 2007;19:366–373.
5. Perentes JY, Abdelnour-Berchtold E, Blatter J. Vacuum-assisted closure device for the management of infected postpneumonectomy chest cavities. *J Thorac Cardiovasc Surg.* 2015;149(3):745–750.
6. Mazzella A, Pardolesi A, Maisonneuve P, et al. Bronchopleural fistula after pneumonectomy: risk factors and management, focusing on open-window thoracostomy. *Semin Thorac Cardiovasc Surg.* 2018;30(1):104–113.
7. Seo H, Kim TJ, Jin KN, et al. Multi-detector row computed tomographic evaluation of bronchopleural fistula: correlation with clinical, bronchoscopic, and surgical findings. *J Comput Assist Tomogr.* 2010;34(1):13–18.
8. Gaur P, Dunne R, Colson YL, et al. Bronchopleural fistula and the role of contemporary imaging. *J Thorac Cardiovasc Surg.* 2014;148(1):341–347.
9. Bribriesco A, Patterson GA. Management of postpneumonectomy bronchopleural fistula: from thoracoplasty to transsternal closure. *Thorac Surg Clin.* 2018;28(3):323–335.
10. Lois M, Noppen M. Bronchopleural fistulas: an overview of the problem with special focus on endoscopic management. *Chest.* 2005;128(6):3955–3965.

11. Boudaya MS, Smadhi H, Zribi H, et al. Conservative management of postoperative bronchopleural fistulas. *J Thorac Cardiovasc Surg.* 2013;146(3):575–579.
12. De Lima A, Holden V, Gesthalter Y, et al. Treatment of persistent bronchopleural fistula with a manually modified endobronchial stent: a case-report and brief literature review. *J Thorac Dis.* 2018;10(10):5960–5963.
13. Algar FJ, Alvarez A, Aranda JL, et al. Prediction of early bronchopleural fistula after pneumonectomy: a multivariate analysis. *Ann Thorac Surg.* 2001;72(5):1662–1667.
14. Deschamps C, Bernard A, Nichols FC, 3rd. et al. Empyema and bronchopleural fistula after pneumonectomy: factors affecting incidence. *Ann Thorac Surg.* 2001;72(1):243–247.
15. Zakkar M, Kanagasabay R, Hunt I. No evidence that manual closure of the bronchial stump has a lower failure rate than mechanical stapler closure following anatomical lung resection. *Interact Cardiovasc Thorac Surg.* 2014;18(4):488–493.
16. Di Maio M, Perrone F, Deschamps C, et al. A meta-analysis of the impact of bronchial stump coverage on the risk of bronchopleural fistula after pneumonectomy. *Eur J Cardiothorac Surg.* 2015;48(2):196–200.
17. Maeda H, Kanzaki M, Kikkawa T, et al. Video-assisted thoracoscopic muscle transposition for acute empyema. *J Cardiothorac Surg.* 2015;10:124.
18. Hollaus PH, Lax F, Wurnig PN, et al. Videothoracoscopic debridement of the postpneumonectomy space in empyema. *Eur J Cardiothorac Surg.* 1999;16(3):283–286.
19. Ernst M, Nies C. Thoracoscopic therapy of pleural empyema after pneumonectomy. *Chirurg.* 1999;70(12):1480–1483.
20. Gossot D, Stern JB, Galetta D, et al. Thoracoscopic management of postpneumonectomy empyema. *Ann Thorac Surg.* 2004;78(1):273–276.
21. Wolter A, Scholz T, Diedrichson J, et al. Bronchopleural fistula after pneumonectomy: interdisciplinary surgical closure by an ipsilateral pedicled latissimus dorsi flap supported by video-assisted thoracoscopy. *J Plast Reconstr Aesthet Surg.* 2013;66(11):1600–1603.

CHAPTER 14

Tuberculous Pleural Effusion and Pott Disease

Claudio Sorino ■ Sergio Agati ■ Stefano Negri ■ Giampietro Marchetti

History of Present Illness

A 47-year-old black woman presented to the emergency room with progressive increase of breathlessness, dry cough, and fever. The symptoms had worsened in the past 3 days. She also complained of neck pain that had been present for several months and episodes of palpitations without chest pain.

Past Medical History

The patient was a never-smoker. She had a family history of malignancy (both mother and grandmother with breast cancer). She had moved from West Africa (Burkina Faso) to Europe 15 years earlier. The patient suffered from meningitis and acute pericarditis 10 and 2 years, respectively, before the current clinical presentation. She was receiving home therapy with only a beta-blocker (bisoprolol 1.25 mg two times daily).

Physical Examination and Early Clinical Findings

The patient had a fever (38.5° C [101.3° F]) and tachycardia (heart rate 129 beats/min). Her oxygen saturation (SpO$_2$) was 94% while at rest and breathing in ambient air. Arterial blood gas (ABG) analysis showed hypoxemia with pH 7.46, partial pressure of oxygen (PaO$_2$) 65.4 mm Hg, and partial pressure of carbon dioxide (PaCO$_2$) 31.5 mm Hg.

Blood pressure was 130/90 mm Hg. Physical examination revealed absence of respiratory sounds in the entire left hemithorax, with dullness on percussion and decreased tactile fremitus.

Chest radiography revealed massive left pleural effusion, with significant contralateral shift of the trachea and the mediastinum (Fig. 14.1). On chest ultrasonography, the pleural effusion was visible over six intercostal spaces along the posterior axillary line. The effusion was not loculated, although it contained minimal fibrinous strands (Fig. 14.2).

Blood tests showed an increase in inflammation indices (C-reactive protein [CRP]: 222.2 mg/L; normal values < 5 mg/L), normal white blood cell (WBC) count (6,810 cells/μL) and normal differential count.

Discussion Topic

The patient has a massive pleural effusion. Let's call the thoracic surgeon; this is something he can sink his teeth into!

ER doctor

Continued

Discussion Topic—cont'd

Thoracic surgeon

The mediastinum is displaced, and the patient is breathless. The liquid must be drained urgently.

ER doctor

Do you prefer to perform only thoracentesis and leave some fluid in the pleural cavity? This would facilitate subsequent diagnostic procedures, such as thoracoscopy.

Thoracic surgeon

The effusion is copious; it would be better to immediately place a chest drain. Moreover, the patient probably has an infection. The analysis of the liquid may provide information on the etiology.

Pulmonologist

Because she immigrated from an area endemic for tuberculosis, we must also investigate it.

Thoracic surgeon

I agree. However, let's not neglect the hypothesis of malignancy. The patient has a family history of cancer.

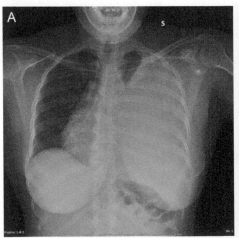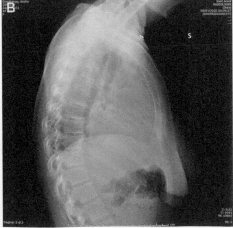

Fig. 14.1 Posteroanterior (A) and lateral (B) chest radiographs showing a massive left pleural effusion with important contralateral deviation of the trachea and the mediastinum.

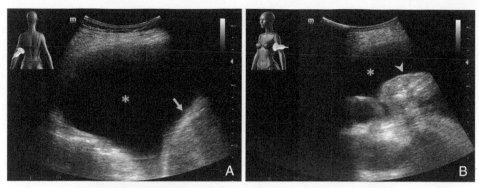

Fig. 14.2   Scan from chest ultrasonography with convex probe showing a large left pleural effusion *(asterisks)*. A flattened diaphragmatic dome *(arrow)* is evident in the transverse scan along the posterior axillary line (A). The longitudinal scan along the midaxillary line shows atelectasis of the whole lung and visible hilum *(arrowhead)*, as occurs in massive pleural effusions (B).

Clinical course

While the patient was still in the emergency room, the thoracic surgeon placed a large-bore chest tube (24-French [Fr]) in the sixth left intercostal space. About 1500 mL of yellowish pleural fluid was immediately evacuated. The tube was then clamped for 2 hours, and then 1400 mL more fluid was gradually drained (at a rate of about 500 mL every 60 minutes). Subsequent chest radiography showed reduction of the left pleural effusion and no more mediastinum shift (Fig. 14.3).

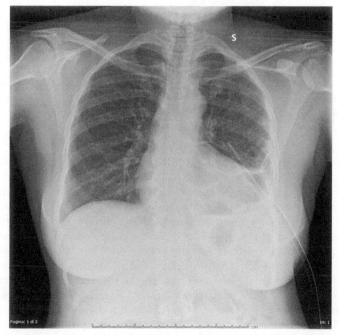

Fig. 14.3   Chest radiograph obtained after pleural drain placement showing reduction of the left pleural effusion and no mediastinal shift.

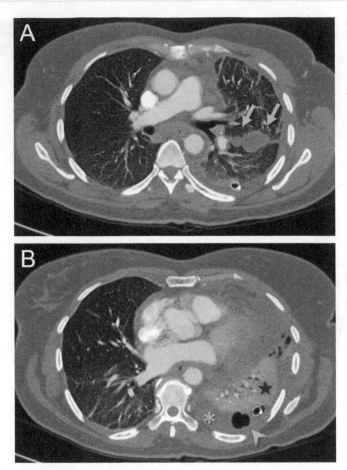

Fig. 14.4 Axial computed tomography (CT) scan (A and B) obtained after chest tube placement showing residual left pleural effusion *(asterisk)* with air content inside *(arrowhead)* and a consolidation in the lower lung lobe with air bronchogram *(star)*. Thickening of the major fissure and intrafissural fluid collections were also evident *(arrows)*.

Echocardiography showed normal left ventricular ejection fraction and no evident pericardial effusion.

The patient was admitted to the pulmonology unit. Empiric antibiotic therapy was initiated (piperacillin/tazobactam 4 g/0.5 g intravenously every 8 hours). Urinary antigen tests for *Pneumococcus* and *Legionella* were negative. No growth was observed on blood cultures.

CT pulmonary angiography (Fig. 14.4) did not show pulmonary embolism. There was a residual left pleural effusion with an air bubble of about 20 mm inside. CT also documented thickening of the major fissure, intrafissural fluid, and a large area of parenchymal hyperdensity with air bronchogram in the left lower lung lobe. In the mediastinum, several oval-shaped lymph nodes were found (maximum thickness of about 8 mm). Moreover, an enlarged internal mammary lymph node was found (Fig. 14.5, A), which was also visible on chest ultrasonography (see Fig. 14.5, B).

Subdiaphragmatic CT showed a left renal cortical lesion of approximately 40 × 37 mm (Fig. 14.6). It had no calcification, and after the injection of the contrast medium, it had density

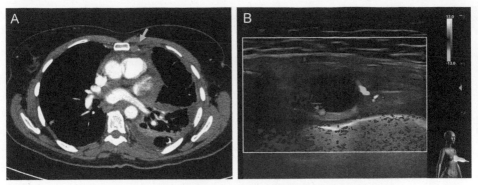

Fig. 14.5 Chest computed tomography (CT) scan in the mediastinal window (A) and scan from chest ultrasonography with linear probe (B) showing an enlarged internal mammary lymph node.

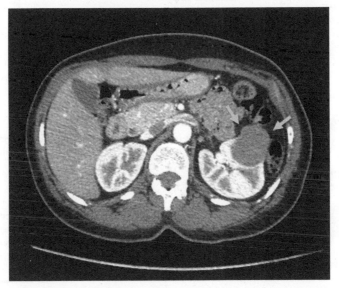

Fig. 14.6 Subdiaphragmatic computed tomography (CT) scan showing a solid left renal cortical lesion.

lower than that of the surrounding parenchyma. These findings suggested a solid lesion probably caused by oncocytoma.

After the pleural fluid evacuation, the patient experienced relief from dyspnea, SpO_2 increased to 97% in ambient air, and CRP decreased to 64 g/dL in a week. However, cough, weakness, and a low-grade fever persisted.

The pleural fluid was a lymphocyte-predominant exudate with lactate dehydrogenase (LDH) 648 units/L, proteins 5.6 g/dL, glucose 70 mg/dL, lymphocytes 75%, and eosinophils 3%. Cultures yielded no growth, and cytological examination did not found malignant cells. The results of both microscopy and analysis of ribosomal RNA of *Mycobacterium tuberculosis* complex (MTC) with ribosomal ribonucleic acid–polymerase chain reaction (rRNA-PCR) on pleural fluid were negative.

Discussion Topic

Pulmonologist

The differential diagnosis of lymphocyte-predominant effusions includes malignancy and tuberculosis.

Thoracic surgeon

Yet we didn't found malignant cells or mycobacteria in the pleural fluid.

Infectious disease specialist

Direct examination of pleural fluid for acid-fast bacilli in immunocompetent individuals is not recommended because the result is usually negative unless the patient has tuberculous empyema.

Pulmonologist

The enlarged internal mammary lymph node can be a sentinel sign of tuberculous pleurisy. Wasn't a QuantiFERON test performed?

Infectious disease specialist

Yes, we're waiting for the result. Most likely the QuantiFERON result will be positive because of the patient's country of origin. However, this doesn't indicate active infection.

Pulmonologist

I agree, it just allows us to verify that the patient came into contact with *Mycobacterium tuberculosis*. In this clinical context, a positive QuantiFERON result would indicate very high suspicion of TB. We should examine other specimens, such as sputum, gastric aspirate, and bronchoalveolar lavage.

The result of interferon-gamma (IFN-γ) release assay (QuantiFERON-TB Gold) was positive (9.75 units/mL; normal values < 0.20). Subsequently, bronchoscopy was performed. This revealed no intrabronchial lesions. The bronchial mucosa was diffusely hyperemic and easily bleeding on contact with the bronchoscope tube. Mucus was present throughout the bronchial tree, especially in the left lower lobar bronchus. Here bronchoalveolar lavage (BAL) was performed.

Direct microscopic examination and search for the genetic material of *M. tuberculosis* by rRNA-PCR were negative. The search for malignant tumor cells was negative as well. The culture results for BAL fluid were positive for *Enterobacter cloacae* and *Candida albicans,* both with low colony counts (1000 colony-forming units [CFU]/mL).

The pleural drainage was inactive for greater than 72 hours, and the patient complained of pain in the insertion site. Therefore the chest tube was removed.

Because of persistence of neck pain, the patient underwent cervical spine CT, which documented erosion in the body of the second cervical vertebra (C2) with posterior displacement of the odontoid process and reduction of the spinal canal space. The patient was evaluated by a

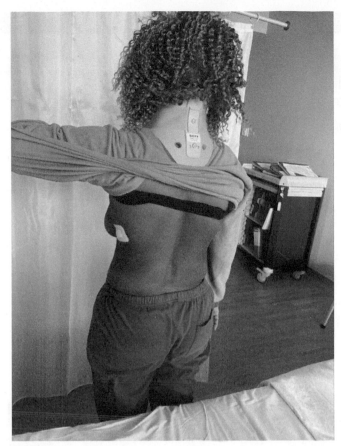

Fig. 14.7 Photo of the patient wearing Philadelphia neck collar. A patch is still present at the site of entry of the chest tube into the chest.

neurosurgeon, who ordered the use of a Philadelphia-type collar (Fig. 14.7) and recommended magnetic resonance imaging (MRI) of the cervical spine. This confirmed the lesion in C2 but did not allow determining whether it was caused by malignancy or infection (Fig. 14.8).

Discussion Topic

Infectious disease specialist

Too many elements lead to this diagnosis of tuberculosis (TB). The spine is one of the areas of extrapulmonary localization of TB. I would initiate empirical therapy even without identifying the mycobacterium.

Thoracic surgeon

I don't agree. None of the investigations confirmed the diagnosis of TB. Who says the patient has concurrent TB and cancer? It is necessary to obtain a definitive diagnosis, and we haven't yet used all the options.

Continued

Discussion Topic—cont'd

Pulmonologist

I think total body positron emission tomography (PET) will be useful, too. It can provide more information on the cervical spine lesion, the renal mass, and other possible disease localization.

Thoracic surgeon

I recommend medical or surgical thoracoscopy.

Pulmonologist

There may be adhesions that hinder the procedure.

Thoracic surgeon

You should be able to lyse the adhesions and perform biopsies.

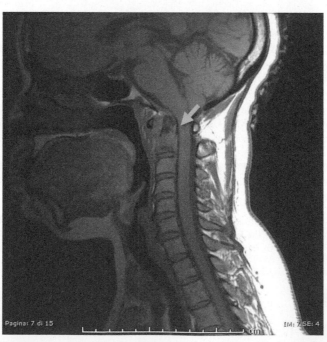

Fig. 14.8 Magnetic resonance imaging (MRI) of the cervical spine showing extensive damage to the second cervical vertebra.

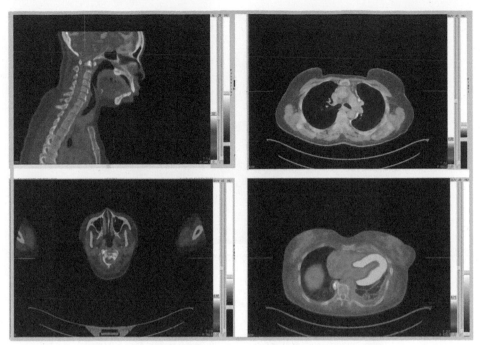

Fig. 14.9 Positron emission tomography (PET) images. Fluorodeoxyglucose (FDG) uptake was found in the left lower pleura, the right pleuropulmonary paravertebral area, the left internal mammary lymph node, some subcarinal and hilar lymph nodes, and the second cervical vertebra.

The patient underwent positron emission tomography (PET; Fig. 14.9), which showed an intense and widespread fluorodeoxyglucose (FDG) uptake in the left lower pleura, with maximum standard uptake value (SUV_{max}) of 9.6. A further focal uptake was visible in the right pleuropulmonary paravertebral area (near D8-D9; SUV_{max} 12.4), the left internal mammary lymph node, and some small subcarinal and hilar lymph nodes. The lesion in the cervical vertebra had an intense FDG uptake as well (SUV_{max} 13.4). In contrast, the left kidney mass did not show a significant FDG uptake. PET findings were highly suggestive of tuberculous pleurisy with extrapulmonary involvement, although these findings could not exclude malignancies.

Medical thoracoscopy was proposed. Signed informed consent was obtained from the patient. She was positioned in the lateral decubitus position, with the affected side up. The patient breathed spontaneously with slight supplemental oxygen via nasal cannula. Blood pressure, electrocardiography (ECG) values, and oxygen saturation were monitored. Moderate sedation was achieved with fentanyl and midazolam. Ultrasonography was used to evaluate the best entry site. Local anesthetic (2% lidocaine) was injected into the skin, subcutaneous tissue, adjacent ribs, and parietal pleura. A small incision was made in the seventh intercostal space at the midaxillary line. An 8-mm trocar was inserted, residual fluid was gently aspirated, and a semirigid pleuroscope was introduced into the pleural space. The entire pleural cavity was explored with evidence of pleural hyperemia with multiple nodules and some pleural adhesions (Fig. 14.10). In the suspected areas, parietal pleural biopsies were performed with flexible forceps under direct vision. At the end of the procedure, a 24-Fr chest tube was placed and maintained for a few days. Histology of parietal pleural biopsies showed granulomas with epithelioid cell (Langerhans giant cells) and caseous necrosis (Fig. 14.11). This confirmed the diagnosis of tuberculous pleurisy.

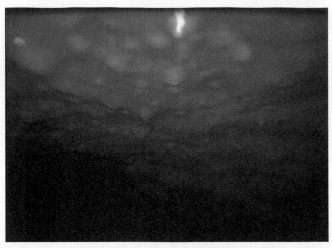

Fig. 14.10 Medical thoracoscopy. Direct vision of parietal pleural hyperemia with multiple nodules.

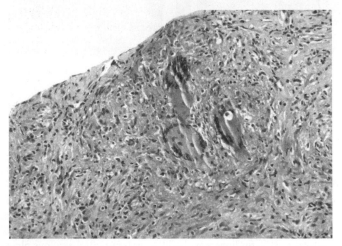

Fig. 14.11 Histology of parietal pleural biopsies (hematoxylin-eosin staining; magnification ×200) showing epithelioid cell granulomas with focal caseous necrosis.

Recommended Therapy and Further Indications at Discharge

The patient was discharged with the diagnosis of "tuberculosis (TB) with pleural and cervical spine involvement." Anti-TB treatment was initiated with the four-drug regimen (rifampicin, isoniazid, pyrazinamide, and ethambutol) and concomitant administration of pyridoxine (vitamin B_6).

Monthly outpatient visits at the infectious disease department were scheduled.

Follow-Up and Outcomes

The patient remained afebrile and experienced progressive improvement of cough and dyspnea. Chest radiography performed 1 month after discharge showed slight elevation of the left hemidiaphragm and blunting of the costophrenic angle (Fig. 14.12). After 2 months of antituberculosis

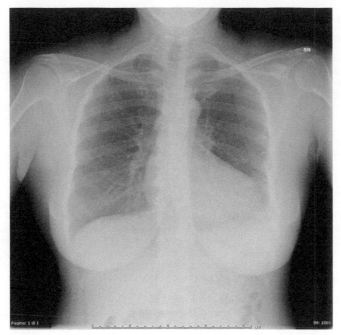

Fig. 14.12 Follow-up chest radiograph showing residual blunting of the left costophrenic angle.

treatment, the therapeutic regimen was modified, and the patient continued to take only rifampicin and isoniazid.

Abdominal MRI confirmed a left solid renal mass, and nephrectomy was scheduled by the urologist.

Focus On

Diagnostic Workup of Suspected Tuberculous Pleural Effusion

The diagnosis of tuberculous pleural effusion (TPE) requires demonstration of *Mycobacterium tuberculosis* (MTB) in biological specimens (e.g., sputum, pleural fluid, pleural biopsy) or epithelioid cells and/or caseating granulomas in the parietal pleura, even in the absence of acid-fast bacilli. Granulomas without caseous necrosis may occur in other diseases, such as fungal infections, sarcoidosis, tularemia, rheumatoid pleuritis, and some vasculitides, although greater than 95% of patients with granulomatous pleuritis have tuberculosis (TB). High values of biomarkers, such as adenosine deaminase or interferon-gamma (IFN-γ) in the pleural fluid can indicate a presumptive diagnosis in the appropriate clinical context.

Thoracentesis enables evaluation of the characteristics of pleural fluid and aid in the differential diagnosis. However, it has a marginal role in the diagnosis of tuberculous pleuritis. Indeed, the smear of pleural fluid is rarely positive, whereas MTB grows only in 20% to 40% of pleural fluid cultures and requires several weeks. Nucleic acid amplification tests (NAATs) on pleural fluid are very rapid but have only slightly higher sensitivity (30%–50%). Thus a negative NAAT result does not rule out tuberculous pleurisy.

Closed biopsies of the parietal pleura, under guidance of ultrasonography or CT, can be used as the primary diagnostic procedure in patients with pleural thickening.

Thoracoscopy can be used if closed pleural biopsies fail to provide a diagnosis or if the patient has pleural effusion either without evident pleural thickening or with previously known benign pleural diseases. Overall, thoracoscopy has a diagnostic yield of nearly 100% and also allows for washing the pleural cavity, thus helping lung reexpansion. It is a very safe procedure, with rates of major and minor complications of 1% and 10%, respectively. Under direct visualization, tuberculous pleurisy typically appears as parietal pleura with patchy inflammation, extensively covered by multiple granulomas. Adhesions are also often present, especially at the level of the costodiaphragmatic recess.

Focus On

Overview of Tuberculosis Treatment

Patients who have been diagnosed with active pulmonary tuberculosis (TB) and have not received anti-tuberculosis drugs for longer than 1 month (the so-called new cases) should be treated for 6 months.

The initial (intensive) phase lasts 2 months and consists of a four-drug regimen with isoniazid, rifampicin, pyrazinamide, and ethambutol.

This regimen quickly kills the tubercle bacilli, and most smear-positive patients become negative within 2 months. However, therapy is extended if the patient has cavitary disease and remains culture positive after 2 months of treatment.

Treatment in the subsequent 4 months, which constitutes the continuation phase, aims to prevent relapse, and consists of only isoniazid plus rifampicin. Continuation therapy can be extended to 9 to 12 months in severe extrapulmonary disease (e.g., in case of neurological involvement).

Patients who have positive results on smear or culture analysis despite previous antituberculosis treatment (retreatment cases) have a higher likelihood of drug resistance. They should be started on a five-drug regimen, which should be modified on the basis of results from drug susceptibility testing.

The term *multidrug-resistant tuberculosis* (MDR-TB) refers to isolates that are resistant to both isoniazid and rifampin and possibly other drugs. The intensive-phase treatment (with at least five drugs) for MDR-TB should be 5 to 7 months, followed by the continuation phase (with at least four drugs) so that the total duration of treatment is 18 to 24 months after culture conversion.

All patients should be closely observed for 2 years after completion of treatment.

Surgical resection of an infected lung can be considered if the prognosis is poor despite medical treatment.

Extensively drug-resistant tuberculosis (XDR-TB) is established by the presence of an isolate that is resistant to isoniazid, rifampin, at least one of the quinolones, and at least one injectable drug. Treatment options for XDR-TB are very limited.

Patients with positive results on tuberculin skin testing or interferon-gamma release assay (IGRA) should receive a course of therapy for latent TB. Different regimens for latent TB are possible (e.g., isoniazid for 6–9 months, or isoniazid plus rifampicin for 3 months). Pyridoxine supplementation is usually ordered during isoniazid therapy to prevent peripheral neuropathy.

Focus On

Extrapulmonary Tuberculosis and Pott Disease

Tuberculosis (TB) typically affects the lungs, but it can also involve other parts of the body. Extrapulmonary TB occurs in about 15% to 20% of subjects with active disease and is more common in immunosuppressed individuals and young children.

It is usually caused by hematogenous dissemination of bacilli from pulmonary lesions or through infection of the genitourinary system. However, the infection can also spread through different mechanisms, such as continuity from an adjacent organ. The main sites involved, in order of frequency, are the lymph nodes, pleura, genitourinary tract, bones and joints, and meninges.

Widespread blood dissemination causes *miliary TB*.

When TB involves bones, it is known as *osseous tuberculosis* and occurs as a form of osteomyelitis. Approximately 10% of patients with extrapulmonary TB have skeletal involvement.

TB of the spine, also known as *Pott disease*, represents the most common form of skeletal TB, accounting for nearly 50% of skeletal TB cases, followed by TB of the hips and knees. It is uncommon in Western countries, where it is usually diagnosed in immigrants coming from TB-endemic areas.

Pott disease mainly affects the lower thoracic and upper lumbar spine. It occurs as a form of spondylitis, with frequent involvement of more than one vertebra because segmental arteries bifurcate to supply two adjacent vertebrae. The vertebral body is more commonly affected compared with the posterior arch.

Typically the infection extends to the intervertebral disk and leads to its destruction, collapse of the vertebral bodies, and anterior wedging. Consequently, kyphosis and distortion of the spinal anatomy develop.

Localized pain is the most common symptom, often associated with muscle spasm and stiffness. It can worsen over weeks and months. After spinal cord compression occurs, progressively worsening neurological deficits can develop, leading up to paraplegia.

Late-onset paraplegia can be related to osteophytes and other chronic degenerative changes at a site of prior infection. Vertebral edema can result from a cold abscess.

Antibiotic therapy is the most important modality and follows standard regimens and principles. Sometimes surgery is needed to decompress the spinal cord.

LEARNING POINTS

- The analysis of pleural effusion cannot exclude the diagnosis of TB.
- Medical thoracoscopy demonstrates high diagnostic accuracy in suspected tuberculous pleural effusion, allowing for direct visualization of the pleura and targeted biopsies.
- *Pott disease* refers to the tuberculous involvement of the spine, usually as a result of hematogenous spread from the lungs or other sites.
- The enlargement of an internal mammary lymph node ipsilateral to pleural effusion is suggestive of tuberculous pleurisy.

Further Reading

1. Wang Z, Xu LL, Wu YB, et al. Diagnostic value and safety of medical thoracoscopy in tuberculous pleural effusion. *Respir Med.* 2015;109(9):1188–1192.
2. Light RW. Update on tuberculous pleural effusion. *Respirology.* 2010;15(3):451–458.
3. Vorster MJ, Allwood BW, Diacon AH, Koegelenberg CF. Tuberculous pleural effusions: advances and controversies. *J Thorac Dis.* 2015;7(6):981–991.
4. Porcel JM. Advances in the diagnosis of tuberculous pleuritis. *Ann Transl Med.* 2016;4(15):282.
5. Agarwal R, Aggarwal AN, Gupta D. Diagnostic accuracy and safety of semirigid thoracoscopy in exudative pleural effusions: a meta-analysis. *Chest.* 2013;144(6):1857–1867.
6. Shaikh F, Lentz R, Feller-Kopman D, Maldonado F. Medical thoracoscopy in the diagnosis of pleural disease: a guide for the clinician. *Expert Rev Respir Med.* 2020.
7. Messineo L, Quadri F, Valsecchi A, et al. Internal mammary lymph node visualization as a sentinel sonographic sign of tuberculous pleurisy. *Ultraschall Med.* 2019;40(4):488–494 [in German].

PART III

Miscellanea

Miscellanea

CHAPTER 15

Cloudy Pleural Effusion in a Heavy Smoker With Rheumatoid Arthritis

Michele Mondoni ■ Paolo Carlucci ■ Claudio Sorino ■ Giampietro Marchetti ■ David Feller-Kopman

History of Present Illness

A 60-year-old Caucasian man was referred to our pulmonology clinic with a 1-month history of dyspnea and bilateral symmetrical arthralgias, mostly in the metacarpophalangeal joints and wrists. Chest radiography revealed right-sided pleural effusion without any lung parenchymal involvement (Fig. 15.1).

Past Medical History

The patient had worked as a bricklayer and was a current heavy smoker (50 pack-year smoking history). He had a 9-year history of rheumatoid arthritis, which was being treated with methotrexate (15 mg/wk) and prednisone (10 mg/day). He denied any alcohol abuse.

Physical Examination and Early Clinical Findings

At admission, the patient was afebrile, oxygen saturation measured by pulse oximetry was 97% on room air, heart rate was 72 beats/min, and blood pressure was 125/75 mm Hg.

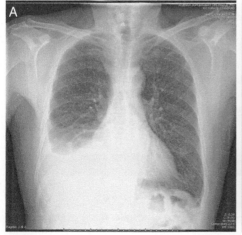
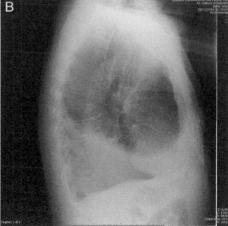

Fig. 15.1 Chest radiograph (A: anteroposterior; B: lateral) showing right-sided pleural effusion without lung parenchymal abnormalities.

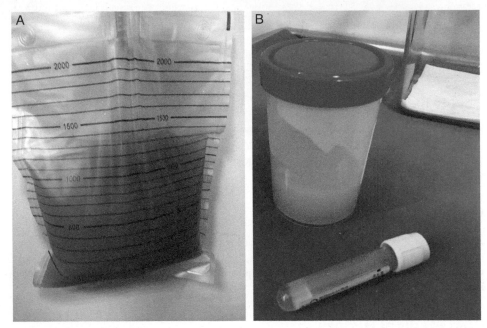

Fig. 15.2 Turbid appearance of the pleural effusion drained by performing thoracentesis. A: drainage bag; B: container and test tube with samples for analysis.

Physical examination revealed decreased breath sounds, decreased tactile fremitus, and dullness to percussion in the right lower pulmonary field. Bilateral swelling was evident in all the proximal interphalangeal and metacarpophalangeal joints of the hands and in the wrists.

Chest ultrasonography showed hypoechoic pleural effusion without any significant septation. Routine blood tests showed mild leukocytosis (white blood cell (WBC) count: 12,710/mm³) with a normal differential count, associated to a slight increase in the inflammation indices (C-reactive protein [CRP]: 27.3 mg/L, normal values < 5 mg/L; erythrocytes sedimentation rate [ESR]: 38 mm/h, normal values < 22 mm/h). The electrolyte concentration values and the liver and kidney function test results were unremarkable.

Clinical Course

Ultrasound-guided right thoracentesis was performed, and 1300 mL of cloudy nonmalodorous pleural fluid was drained (Fig. 15.2). The procedure was well tolerated, and the pleural fluid was sent to the laboratory for analysis. The pleural fluid characteristics, which were measured by using a blood gas analyzer in the pulmonology ward, were available in a few minutes: pH 7.11, glucose 23 mg/dL.

Discussion Topic

The patient is immunosuppressed. The gross appearance of the pleural fluid is cloudy, and it has low pH and low glucose concentration. This is an empyema, isn't it?

Pulmonologist A

Discussion Topic—cont'd

Pulmonologist B

I'm not sure that's it. The patient does not have clinical signs of an acute pleural infection, and chest ultrasonography does not show pleural loculation. Moreover, the pleural fluid is nonmalodorous as it would be in the case of an anaerobic infection.

Pulmonologist C

The patient has a known rheumatoid arthritis; that is a cause of pseudochylothorax.

Pulmonologist A

Can pseudochylothorax in rheumatoid arthritis be similar to complicated pleural effusion?

Pulmonologist C

Yes, of course. It usually has a low pH, low glucose, and high lactate dehydrogenase (LDH).

Pulmonologist A

However, I think that tuberculosis or other pleural infections should be ruled out. I suggest insertion of a chest tube as soon as possible.

Pulmonologist B

We also should rule out malignancy. Let's not forget he is a heavy smoker.

Pulmonologist C

To me, thoracoscopic pleural biopsy is the best way to diagnose underlying disease.

In the subsequent days, biochemistry analyses revealed the presence of an exudative effusion (pleural fluid lactate dehydrogenase [LDH]: 805 units/L; serum LDH 401 units, ratio 2.0; pleural fluid protein 3.6 g/dL; and serum protein 3 g/dL, ratio 1.2). Culture of the pleural fluid yielded no growth. Smear microscopy and XpertMTB/RIF results were negative. The cytological analysis showed lymphocytosis (65% of lymphocytes) without malignant cells. Because of the gross appearance of the fluid, further analysis was requested. Triglyceride concentration was low (26 mg/dL) and no chylomicrons were detected. Cholesterol concentration was 247 mg/dL. The cholesterol/triglyceride ratio was 9.5. Cholesterol crystals were absent. On the basis of these findings, a diagnosis of pseudochylothorax was made.

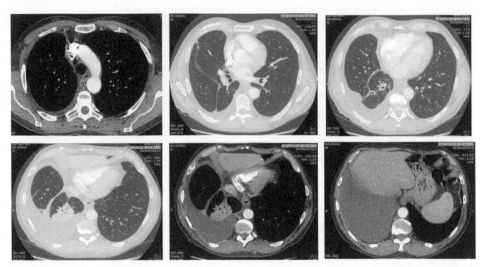

Fig. 15.3 Axial chest computed tomography (CT) scans, obtained after thoracentesis, showing thickened parietal pleura on the right, free right pleural effusion, and segmental atelectasis in the right lower lobe. No further parenchymal abnormalities are present.

Other laboratory investigations were then requested: human immunodeficiency virus (HIV), hepatitis C virus (HCV), and hepatitis B virus (HBV) serological test results were unremarkable. The QuantiFERON-TB test result was positive.

Chest computed tomography (CT), performed after thoracentesis, showed the presence of thickened parietal pleura on the right, small-to-moderate residual right pleural effusion, and segmental atelectasis in the right lower lobe. Any other parenchymal abnormalities and mediastinal lymph node enlargement were not detected (Fig. 15.3).

Because of the presence of pseudochylothorax of unknown etiology in a heavy smoker with rheumatoid arthritis and long-term immunosuppressive therapy, pleural biopsy was scheduled.

The patient underwent medical thoracoscopy, under local anesthesia (lidocaine) and moderate sedation (intravenous midazolam and fentanyl). The thoracoscopic investigation confirmed the presence of cloudy pleural fluid, which was immediately drained (1000 mL) (Fig. 15.4).

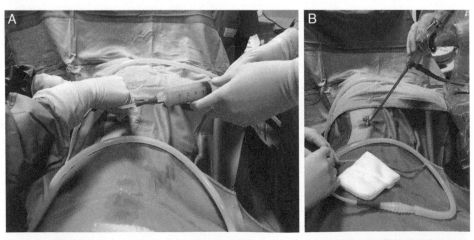

Fig. 15.4 Medical thoracoscopy. A: cloudy pleural effusion drained just before insertion of the thoracoscope; B: inspection of the pleural cavity.

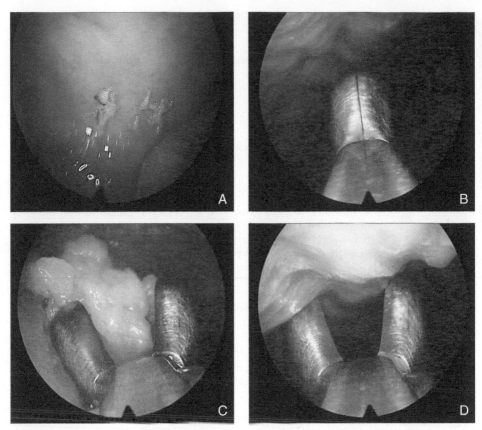

Fig. 15.5 Thoracoscopic examination showing soft yellow peel over the basal parietal pleura (A). The parietal pleura appears thickened and rough in the upper two-thirds of the chest cavity (B). Multiple biopsy specimens of both the yellow material (C) and the parietal pleura (D) were obtained.

Endoscopic examination revealed soft yellow peel over both the basal parietal and the visceral pleura associated with the presence of fibrin deposit in the thoracic cavity. In the upper two-thirds, the parietal pleura was thickened and rough. Multiple biopsy specimens were obtained from both the parietal pleura and fibrin for histopathological and microbiological examinations (Fig. 15.5).

Discussion Topic

Pulmonologist A

Could talc pleurodesis during medical thoracoscopy be useful to reduce the risk of relapse of pleural effusion?

Pulmonologist B

Pleurodesis is controversial in benign effusion, and current endoscopic findings do not suggest malignancy. Moreover, pleurodesis is contraindicated in the case of tuberculous pleurisy, and we have not yet ruled it out.

Continued

Discussion Topic—cont'd

Pulmonologist C

Furthermore, computed tomography (CT) has indicated that the lung may be partially trapped: pleurodesis would be difficult to obtain. An indwelling pleural catheter should be considered.

Pulmonologist A

And what about pleurectomy and decortication? Under what circumstances can they be useful?

Pulmonologist B

In the case of relapsing pleural fluid and persistent symptoms (i.e., dyspnea) despite treatment of underlying disease, pleurectomy with decortication could be considered to obtain full expansion of the lung; however, we should discuss its risks and benefits with the patient.

Microbiological tests on the pleural fluid all yielded negative results, demonstrating no growth of bacteria or *Mycobacterium tuberculosis* (MTB). Nested polymerase chain reaction (PCR) of both the parietal pleura and fibrin showed negative results for the presence of deoxyribonucleic acid (DNA) of MTB. Histological examination of pleural biopsy specimens showed infiltration by inflammatory cells, multinucleated giant cells, and very few mesothelial cells, in a background of amorphous material (i.e., fibrin). No malignant cells or granulomas were detected (Fig. 15.6).

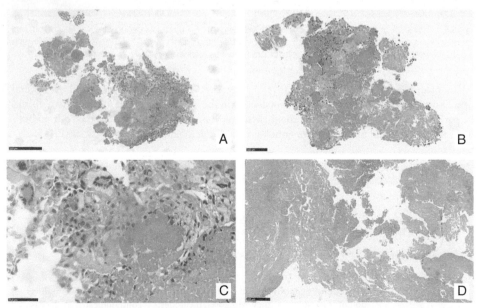

Fig. 15.6 Histopathological examination of the thoracoscopic pleural biopsies showing acute and chronic pleural inflammation (A, B), multinucleated giant cells (C), and very few mesothelial cells in a background of amorphous material (i.e., fibrin) (D). No malignant cells or granulomas are present.

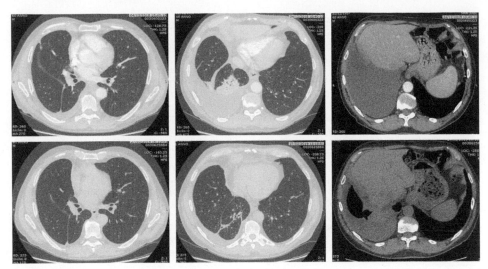

Fig. 15.7 Chest computed tomography (CT) scan obtained before (A–C) and 3 weeks after (D–F) the hospital discharge. CT scans obtained after the discharge show decrease of pleural effusion and partial reduction of the lower lobe segmental atelectasis.

Although a clear rheumatoid nodule was not observed, these findings were highly suspicious of a rheumatoid pleurisy.

On the basis of all of the clinical, laboratory, and instrumental findings, pseudochylothorax in uncontrolled rheumatoid arthritis was the final diagnosis.

Discharge, Follow-Up, and Outcomes

The postoperative course was uneventful, and the patient was discharged from the hospital, after which he started a new treatment for his rheumatoid arthritis (baricitinib, an oral, once-daily selective Janus kinase inhibitor), which resulted in progressive reduction of rheumatoid symptoms in the hands and wrists. Three weeks after discharge, the patient underwent chest ultrasonography and CT, which showed significant reduction in pleural effusion and in the basal lung atelectasis (Fig. 15.7).

Focus On

Pseudochylothorax

Pseudochylothorax (PCT), also called *cholesterol effusion*, is a rare form of pleural effusion and it is characterized by high cholesterol concentration. As a result of the high lipid content, chylothorax and PCT have similar gross appearances, with milky or cloudy fluid. However, they have very different etiologies, pathogenesis, and clinical presentations.

In greater than 85% of cases, the etiology of PCT is tuberculosis or rheumatoid arthritis. Other causes include parasitic infections (e.g., echinococcosis and paragonimiasis), yellow nail syndrome, traumas, and malignancies, although it may be associated with any type of chronic effusion, such as those occurring after coronary artery bypass surgery.

It is believed that pleural thickening, occurring in some chronic inflammatory disorders, may block drainage of fluids to the pleural wall lymphatic systems. Cholesterol and lecithin–globulin complexes, released by erythrocytes and neutrophils that undergo lysis in the pleural fluid, consequently become trapped in the pleural cavity.

Continued

Focus On—cont'd

However, about one-fifth of cholesterol pleural effusions occurs without pleural thickening. Thus other unknown pathogenic mechanisms must be involved.

Most of patients with PCT have a history of long-standing pleural disease (months or years) and present with insidious onset of dyspnea. Symptoms of underlying diseases (e.g., weight loss, fever, arthralgias, etc.) are sometimes present. Diagnosis is mainly based on the pleural fluid analysis. In the majority of cases, PCTs are exudates with both high lactate dehydrogenase (LDH) levels (often > 800 units/L, caused by pleural space inflammation) and high protein content (often > 3 g/dL, caused by increased capillary permeability or lymphatic dysregulation). They usually have a low count of nucleated cells (< 5000 cells/mm^3) and are lymphocyte predominant. The pleural fluid cholesterol level is greater than 200 mg/dL, whereas the triglyceride level is less than 50 mg/dL, with a cholesterol/triglyceride ratio less than 1. Although not always present, cholesterol crystals are virtually diagnostic of cholesterol effusion. Chylomicrons, which are pathognomonic of chylothorax, are absent.

Clinical findings and results of laboratory tests, chest imaging, and pleural biopsies may contribute to the diagnosis of the underlying pathology.

The management of pseudochylothorax is based on a sequential approach, and the outcome is favorable in the majority of the cases. Treating the underlying disease is essential. In case of symptomatic pleural effusions, repeated thoracentesis or chest tube/indwelling pleural catheter placement is indicated. In the presence of symptomatic trapped lung, decortication or pleurectomy may be necessary.

Focus On

Pleural Fluid pH Measurement

Pleural fluid pH measurement is important in the management of patients with exudative pleural effusions. Common variations in the method used to obtain pleural fluid specimens affect the accuracy of the value obtained.

Pleural fluid pH measured by a blood gas analyzer is the only recommended method to obtain an accurate evaluation. Pleural fluid pH is decreased by exposure to acidic fluids, such as local anesthetic or heparin retained in the syringe or injected into the pleural cavity. In contrast, exposure of the sample to air leads to an increase in pH. If immediate analysis is not possible, delay of up to 4 hours does not cause a significant change in pH, even when the sample is kept at room temperature.

Physicians should be aware of their laboratory's method of measurement and only rely on a blood gas analyzer.

The aforementioned factors have less effect on glucose concentration, which may be used to guide management if an accurate pH value is not available.

Focus On

Moderate Sedation in Medical Thoracoscopy

Medical thoracoscopy is a minimally invasive endoscopic procedure for exploration of the pleural cavity and can be performed with the patient placed under moderate sedation and local anesthesia. Bolus administration of fentanyl and midazolam is the preferred method to obtain sedation during the procedure. Although propofol has been shown to be safe for sedation during flexible bronchoscopy, it is not the drug of choice for sedation during medical thoracoscopy. Indeed, studies comparing midazolam and propofol (given either as a bolus or as an infusion) found that the latter is associated with increased risk of adverse events or complications, such as desaturation and hypotension, during medical thoracoscopy. The diagnostic yield of medical thoracoscopy is greater than 95%, and complications are quite rare.

LEARNING POINTS

- When milky or cloudy pleural effusion is found, measurement of cholesterol, triglycerides, and chylomicron concentrations allows for differentiating chylothorax from pseudochylothorax.
- Distinguishing pseudochylothorax from chylothorax is mandatory for the proper management of the underlying disease.
- Tuberculosis and rheumatoid arthritis account for greater than 85% of the causes of pseudochylothorax.
- When pseudochylothorax is found, pleural biopsies are often necessary to identify the etiology.
- To obtain accurate pleural fluid pH measurements, it is essential to use a blood gas analyzer.

Further Reading

1. Kampolis CF, Vlachoyiannopoulos PG. Pseudochylothorax in a patient with rheumatoid arthritis. *J Rheumatol*. 2019;46(2):213–214.
2. Wrightson JM, Stanton AE, Maskell NA, et al. Pseudochylothorax without pleural thickening. Time to reconsider pathogenesis. *Chest*. 2009;136(4):1144–1147.
3. Lama A, Ferreiro L, Toubes ME, et al. Characteristics of patients with pseudochylothorax-a systematic review. *J Thorac Dis*. 2016;8(8):2093–2101.
4. Clinical presentation, diagnosis and management of cholesterol effusion. ©UpToDate 2019, Inc. and/or its affiliates. Available at: www.uptodate.com.
5. Garcia-Zamalloa A. Pseudochylothorax, an unknown disease. *Chest*. 2010;137(4):1004–1005.
6. Avnon LS, Abu-Shakra M, Flusser D, Heimer D, Sion-Vardy N. Pleural effusion associated with rheumatoid arthritis: what cell predominance to anticipate. *Rheumatol Int*. 2007;27(10):919–925.
7. Casalini AG, Mori PA, Majori M, et al. Pleural tuberculosis: medical thoracoscopy greatly increases the diagnostic accuracy. *ERJ Open Res*. 2018;4(1):2017.
8. Bibby AC, Dorn P, Psallidas I, et al. ERS/EACTS statement on the management of malignant pleural effusions. *Eur Respir J*. 2018;52(1):1800349.
9. Bertolaccini L, Viti A, Paiano S, et al. Indwelling pleural catheters: a clinical option in trapped lung. *Thorac Surg Clin*. 2017;27(1):47–55.
10. Mishra EK, Rahman NM. Factors influencing the measurement of pleural fluid pH. *Curr Opin Pulm Med*. 2009;15(4):353–357.
11. Putnam B, Elahi A, Bowling MR. Do we measure pleural fluid pH correctly. *Curr Opin Pulm Med*. 2013;19(4):357–361.
12. Murthy V, Bessich JL. Medical thoracoscopy and its evolving role in the diagnosis and treatment of pleural disease. *J Thorac Dis*. 2017;9(Suppl 10):S1011–S1021.
13. Grendelmeier P, Tamm M, Jahn K, Pflimlin E, Stolz D. Propofol versus midazolam in medical thoracoscopy: a randomized, noninferiority trial. *Respiration*. 2014;88:126–136.

CHAPTER 16

Calcified Pleural Plaques in a Man With Chronic Obstructive Pulmonary Disease

Claudio Sorino ◾ Stefano Negri ◾ Sergio Agati ◾ David Feller-Kopman

History of Present Illness

A 69-year-old Caucasian man presented with concerns of breathlessness during mild efforts, such as walking on flat ground, and a cough with little sputum for several months. He had no fever, chest pain, or nighttime respiratory symptoms. As suggested by the general practitioner, he underwent chest radiography which revealed bilateral opacities suggesting pleural calcifications (Fig. 16.1). Subsequently, he was referred to the outpatient pulmonology clinic.

Past Medical History

The patient was a former smoker (20–40 cigarettes a day for 30 years), but he had stopped smoking 20 years ago (approximately 45 pack-years). He had no clear recollection of any asbestos exposure, although he worked as a welder and a plumber. He had no previous history of tuberculosis, pleural infection, or effusion, but he stated that he had had pneumonia, which was treated with antibiotics at home, 15 years earlier (no imaging was available).

Moreover, he had a history of prostatic hypertrophy and discectomy for a herniated disk in the lumbar region 10 years before the current presentation.

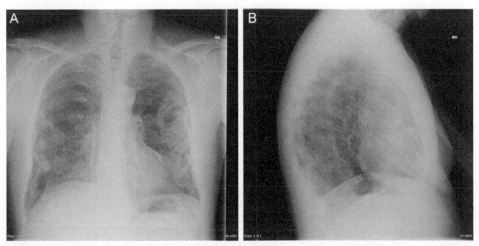

Fig. 16.1 Posteroanterior (A) and lateral (B) chest radiographs showing bilateral irregular opacities caused by calcified pleural plaques.

Physical Examination and Early Clinical Findings

When the patient was at the pulmonology clinic, he was alert and cooperative; was not pale or cyanotic; and had no clubbing, jugular vein distention, or lower limb edema. Breath sounds were slightly reduced, and crackles were audible at the lung bases. Oxygen saturation (SpO_2) measured by pulse oximeter was normal (97% at rest in room air). Simple spirometry showed reduction of the forced expiratory volume in 1 second (FEV_1)/vital capacity (VC) ratio and lowered VC, suggesting a mixed ventilatory defect (obstructive and restrictive). However, lung volumes measured with body plethysmography revealed no reduction in total lung capacity (TLC), whereas residual volume (RV) was increased. These findings were indicative of unique airway obstruction with significant air trapping. A corresponding gas exchange disorder was found, with diffusion capacity for carbon monoxide (DLCO) decreased to 71.2% of the predicted value (Fig. 16.2).

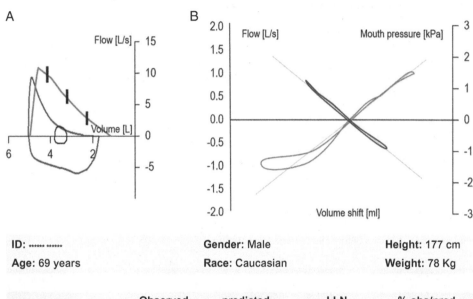

ID: ****** ******   **Gender:** Male   **Height:** 177 cm

Age: 69 years   **Race:** Caucasian   **Weight:** 78 Kg

	Observed	predicted	LLN	% obs/pred
FEV$_1$ (Lit)	1.80	3.22	2.34	58.4
FVC (Lit)	3.11	4.24	3.16	73.3
FEV$_1$/FVC	0.60	0.76	0.63	78.9
Raw (TkPa*s/L)	0.47	0.30	0.30	156.7
RV (Lit)	3.71	2.63	1.96	141.1
TLC (Lit)	7.68	7.06	5.91	108.8
DLCO (ml/min/mmHg)	18.8	26.4	19,7	71.2

Fig. 16.2 Pulmonary function tests. (A) Flow-volume curve. The concavity of the expiratory curve suggests airways obstruction. (B) Plethysmography. The upper intersection angle of the respiratory loops higher than 90 degrees is a sign of airways obstruction. The table shows the measured parameters (post–bronchodilator therapy values). Reduction of FEV$_1$/VC below the lower limit of normal indicates airway obstruction. Reduction in VC and increase in RV are expressions of air-trapping. *DLCO,* diffusing capacity of the lungs for carbon monoxide; *FEV$_1$,* forced expiratory volume in 1 second; *LLN,* lower limit of normal; *RV,* residual volume; *TLC,* total lung capacity; *VC,* vital capacity.

Clinical Course

The patient was diagnosed with chronic obstructive pulmonary disease (COPD). The degree of obstruction was moderate, according to the GOLD guidelines (FEV$_1$ between 50% and 80% of predicted value). The patient was found to have grade 2 dyspnea, according to the Modified Medical Research Council (mMRC) questionnaire. Dual bronchodilator therapy (tiotropium bromide/olodaterol 2.5/2.5 µg, two inhalations once a day) was prescribed, with the main purpose of alleviating symptoms.

Chest computed tomography (CT) was performed (Fig. 16.3), and it revealed extensive bilateral calcified plaques in the parietal, diaphragmatic, and left mediastinal pleurae (adjacent to the

---

Discussion Topic

General practitioner

What do you think of my patient's condition? I saw all those opacities on the chest radiographs.

Pulmonologist

They should be just multiple, extensive, calcified pleural plaques. Viewed en face, they can look like lung lesions.

General practitioner

Yet he claims not to have had any contact with asbestos.

Pulmonologist

Asbestos has been used extensively in the past, and it is found in many materials. Sometimes people don't know they have been exposed to it. However, the radiological findings suggest that he was exposed, probably at work and for a long time.

General practitioner

Do you think those findings are only extrapulmonary ones?

Pulmonologist

It seems so. However, it's prudent to perform chest CT. This can help identify plaques, whether calcified or not, and will allow us to evaluate the lung parenchyma as well.

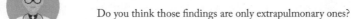

General practitioner

I agree. Asbestos also causes pulmonary fibrosis. Moreover, the patient was a heavy cigarette smoker. His risk for pleural and pulmonary malignancies is much higher than in the general population.

Continued

Discussion Topic—cont'd

Pulmonologist

Pulmonary functional tests have revealed a moderate airway obstruction.
    I have prescribed bronchodilator therapy. I'm sure this will improve his exertional breathlessness.

General practitioner

Should the reduction in diffusion capacity for carbon monoxide (DLCO) suggest the presence of pulmonary interstitium thickening as in asbestosis?

Pulmonologist

Not necessarily. DLCO is commonly reduced in patients with chronic obstructive pulmonary disease (COPD) and emphysema because of loss of alveolar surface available for gas exchange.

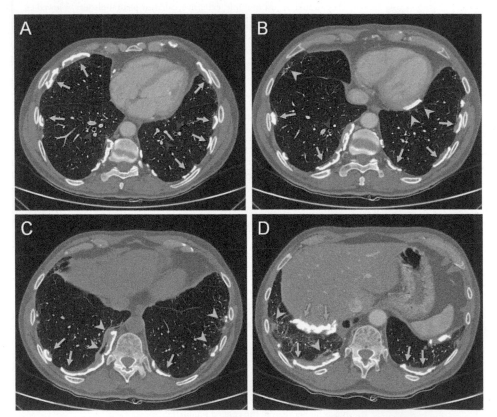

Fig. 16.3 Chest computed tomography (CT) scan showing bilateral calcified plaques in the parietal pleura (A–D, *yellow arrows*), left mediastinal pleura (B, *yellow arrowheads*), and diaphragmatic pleura (D, *blue arrows*). Parenchymal bands (C, D, *green arrowheads*) and bronchiectasis (A, B, *red arrowheads*) are also evident.

pericardial surface). Parenchymal bands in the peripheral region of the lower zones, centrolobular emphysema in the upper lobes, and some bronchiectasis were also evident.

Discussion Topic

General practitioner

Chest computed tomography (CT) has confirmed the presence of pleural plaques.

Pulmonologist A

Pleural thickening or plaques are not a cause for concern. They don't progress to cancer. However, they're an indication of asbestos exposure and thus the patient's high risk for other asbestos-related diseases, including malignant pleural mesothelioma.

General practitioner

Are other investigations required?

Pulmonologist B

In the absence of pleural effusion, I usually don't order further tests. In this case, however, there is a doubtful area in the paravertebral region of the lower right lobe

Pulmonologist A

It's adjacent to a pleural plaque and could be a parenchymal band, which is often an indication of lung asbestosis.
   We could just recommend follow-up with chest CT after 6 months to see if it changes.

Pulmonologist B

I would prefer not to wait and suggest PET to see if the area has active metabolism.

The patient underwent CT/PET, which showed a very small fluorodeoxyglucose (FDG) uptake (maximum standard uptake value [SUV_{max}]: 2.3) corresponding to the peripheral parenchymal bands and, in particular, that of the right lower paravertebral region (Fig. 16.4). The 6-minute walking test and continuous monitoring of nocturnal oxyhemoglobin saturation revealed absence of respiratory failure during effort and sleep, respectively.

Recommended Therapy and Further Indications

The patient was advised to continue the bronchodilator therapy regularly. Pneumococcal and seasonal flu vaccinations were also recommended. Three visits per year at the pneumology outpatient clinic were scheduled.

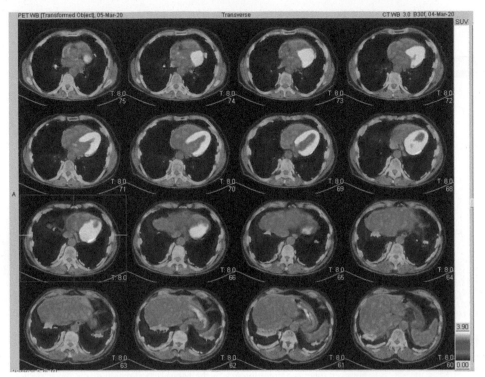

Fig. 16.4 Positron emission tomography (PET) scan showing a very small fluorodeoxyglucose (FDG) uptake (standard uptake value [SUV$_{max}$]: 2.3) corresponding to the peripheral parenchymal bands.

Follow-Up and Outcomes

After 3 months of continuous therapy with bronchodilators, the patient reported improvement in exertional dyspnea. CT/PET after 1 year showed almost unchanged findings, with an even lower FDG uptake (SUV$_{max}$ 2.0) in the peripheral pulmonary bands with FDG uptake.

Focus On

Consequences of Asbestos Exposure

Asbestos is the generic name for six minerals that are found naturally in the environment and that have been used in commercial products for their characteristics, such as strength, flexibility, insulation, and chemical inertness.

Asbestos fibers can float in the air for a long time and can be easily inhaled. They penetrate deep into the respiratory system, to the respiratory bronchioles and the pulmonary alveoli, where they cause an inflammatory response. Alveolar macrophages can phagocytose the asbestos fibers, but not remove them; thus these fibers usually remain in the body for the rest of the exposed person's life.

The diseases caused by asbestos inhalation include fibrotic alteration of the lungs (asbestosis), focal thickening and hardening of the pleura (pleural plaques), benign asbestos pleural effusion (BAPE), lung cancer, and malignant pleural mesothelioma.

Pleural plaques are presumed to be the result of pleural inflammation caused by asbestos fibers transported to the pleural surface along the lymphatic channels and/or through direct penetration.

Calcified pleural plaques usually appear later compared with fibrous plaques and are more often associated with pulmonary parenchymal asbestosis.

Focus On

Pleural Plaques

Pleural plaques are the most common manifestation of asbestos-related disease. These plaques do not progress to malignant pleural mesothelioma; they are localized collagen fiber deposits, typically found in the parietal pleura, most frequently in the lower portions of the chest, and in the mediastinal pleura. Pleural plaques may be calcified; however, most (> 80%) are not. They are usually asymptomatic and are occasionally encountered during routine chest radiography or computed tomography (CT), appearing as localized areas of pleural thickenings. On microscopy, pleural plaques appear as intertwined collagen bundles. Pleural plaques usually manifest greater than 20 years after exposure. Approximately half the individuals exposed to asbestos, even with low-dose and intermittent exposure, develop pleural plaques over time. This differs from asbestosis, which is pulmonary fibrosis occurring only after prolonged and heavy inhalation of asbestos fibers (estimated cumulative exposure of > 25 fibers/mL–years), showing a dose–response relationship between the concentration of fibers in the lungs and the severity or extent of the fibrosis.

Although most of the pleural plaques can be attributed to exposure to asbestos, they have also been found in individuals exposed to only fluoroedenite and erionite fibers.

Plaque-like calcification can also be found in other pathologies, such as granulomatous diseases (e.g., pleural tuberculosis).

Various conditions can mimic pleural plaques, for example, the presence of extrapleural fat, diffuse pleural thickening, and outcomes of hemothorax, rib fractures, and talc pleurodesis.

Primary and secondary pleural malignancies should be considered in the differential diagnosis.

The term *pseudoplaque* usually refers to plaque-like lung opacity that is contiguous with the visceral pleura, formed by small coalescent nodules. This radiological finding can be found in patients with sarcoidosis, silicosis, and coal worker's pneumoconiosis (CWP).

Focus On

Lung Volume Measurement

Spirometry is a basic tool for the evaluation of airway function. It measures displaceable lung volumes (i.e., those that can be inhaled or exhaled). Spirometry identifies bronchial obstruction when the ratio of forced expiratory volume in 1 second (FEV_1) and vital capacity (VC) is below the lower limit of normal (LLN).

However, simple spirometry cannot measure the volume of gas that remains within the lungs after maximal exhalation (residual volume [RV]) and, consequently, total lung capacity (TLC = VC + RV).

If VC is lower than LLN, lung restriction may be suspected. Its confirmation requires evidence of TLC reduction below the LLN. Indeed, reduction in VC can also result from premature airway closure during forced exhalation, as occurs in asthma, or the loss of elastic recoil, as occurs in emphysema. This results in RV increase (air trapping), whereas TLC can be normal or augmented (lung hyperinflation).

Nondisplaceable lung volumes can be measured with special methods, such as body plethysmography, helium gas dilution, and nitrogen washout. Plethysmography measures the total amount of gas present in the thorax, including any trapped gas within the lungs. Conversely, gas dilution and washout techniques measure only the volume of gas in the lungs that is actually in direct communication with the airways and the environment. Thus, they may underestimate TLC if very poorly ventilated airspaces are present.

When plethysmography is performed, flow and oral pressures are plotted against the displaced volume, creating two loops. In the absence of obstruction (healthy individuals or those with restriction), the two loops intersect at an upper angle lower than 90 degrees. In the case of airway obstruction, this angle usually is greater than 90 degrees. If emphysema is present, the respiratory loop takes on a typical club shape.

A mixed pattern of obstructive and restrictive ventilatory defects may occur as a result of the coexistence of an airway disease (e.g., asthma or chronic obstructive pulmonary disease [COPD]) with other parenchymal lung diseases or extrapulmonary disorders (e.g., interstitial lung diseases, congestive heart failure, obesity, previous thoracic surgery, kyphoscoliosis).

LEARNING POINTS

- Pleural plaques can be considered a marker of asbestos exposure.
- Pleural plaques do not progress to malignancy.
- Asbestos-related diseases include pulmonary fibrosis (asbestosis) and malignant pleural mesothelioma.
- Both lung emphysema and asbestosis affect DLCO values.
- Smoking and asbestos exposure significantly increase an individual's risk for pleural and pulmonary malignancies.

Further Reading

1. Criée CP, Sorichter S, Smith HJ, et al. Body plethysmography—its principles and clinical use. *Respir Med.* 2011;105(7):959–971.
2. Cugell DW, Kamp DW. Asbestos and the pleura: a review. *Chest.* 2004;125(3):1103–1117.
3. Graham BL, Steenbruggen I, Miller MR, et al. Standardization of spirometry. 2019 update. An official American Thoracic Society and European Respiratory Society technical statement. *Am J Respir Crit Care Med.* 2019;200(8):e70–e88.
4. Granchelli AM, Liou TG, Kanner R, Sorino C. Lung volumes and further assessment: beyond spirometry. In: Sorino C, ed. *Diagnostic Evaluation of the Respiratory System.*1st ed. New Delhi, India: Jaypee Brothers Medical Publishers; 2017.
5. Kim Y, Myong JP, Lee JK, et al. CT characteristics of pleural plaques related to occupational or environmental asbestos exposure from South Korean asbestos mines. *Korean J Radiol.* 2015;16(5):1142–1152.
6. Preisser AM, Schlemmer K, Herold R, et al. Relations between vital capacity, CO diffusion capacity and computed tomographic findings of former asbestos-exposed patients: a cross-sectional study. *J Occup Med Toxicol.* 2020;15:21.
7. Roach HD, Davies GJ, Attanoos R, et al. Asbestos: when the dust settles an imaging review of asbestos-related disease. *Radiographics.* 2002;22(Spec No):S167–S184.

CHAPTER 17

Middle and Low Back Pain Due to Pulmonary Embolism With Ipsilateral Pleural Effusion

Claudio Sorino ■ Alessandro Squizzato ■ Natalia Buda
■ Giampietro Marchetti ■ David Feller-Kopman

History of Present Illness

A 21-year-old Caucasian woman went to the emergency room complaining of cough, with three episodes of mild hemoptysis. The previous day she had a high fever (40° C [104° F]). Moreover, she had been undergoing physiotherapy for middle and low back pain for a week.

Past Medical History

The patient's past medical history was unremarkable, except for common childhood infectious diseases and pyelonephritis at age 16 years. The patient, who worked as a shop assistant, was thin but with normal physical measurements (height 155 cm, weight 49 kg, body mass index [BMI] = 20.4). She reported smoking a few cigarettes a day and engaging in regular physical activity three times a week. She had been taking a combined estrogen–progestogen oral contraceptive for about 8 months. No previous drug adverse events were reported.

Physical Examination and Early Clinical Findings

The patient was alert, and the temperature had come down to 37.5° C (99.5° F), but she had just taken paracetamol 1000 mg. Physical examination revealed several red circles on the skin of her left back (Fig. 17.1) resulting from undergoing a traditional Chinese massage technique, in which suction cups are used for pain relief (the so-called cupping therapy). Reduction of breath sounds and dullness to percussion at the left lower chest were evident. Oxygen saturation (SpO_2) was 98% in room air, arterial blood gas (ABG) analysis showed normal partial pressure of carbon dioxide ($PaCO_2$ 39 mm Hg) and partial pressure of oxygen (PaO_2 88 mm Hg).

Electrocardiography (ECG) demonstrated sinus tachycardia at 100 beats/min. Chest radiography and ultrasonography showed unilateral left pleural effusion and slight ipsilateral consolidation of the pulmonary parenchyma, with a vascular sign at the margin (Figs. 17.2 and 17.3). Blood tests revealed an increase in inflammatory markers (C-reactive protein [CRP]: 42 mg/L; normal values < 5 mg/L) and leukocytosis (white blood cell [WBC] count: 12,500 cells/μL).

Empirical therapy was begun, including broad-spectrum antibiotics (ceftriaxone 1 g intravenously once a day plus oral azithromycin 500 mg once a day), and analgesics (paracetamol 1 g orally, as needed). The same day the patient was admitted to the pulmonology unit.

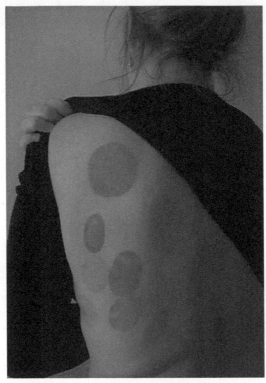

Fig. 17.1 Red marks on the left back caused by a previous attempt at relieving pain by using unconventional therapies ("cupping").

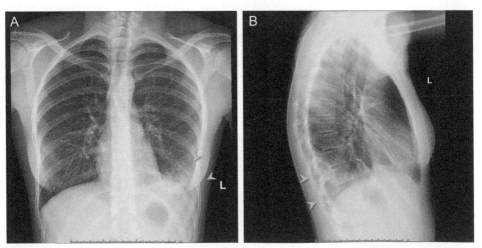

Fig. 17.2 Posteroanterior (A) and lateral (B) chest radiographs showing a small left pleural effusion and patchy areas of decreased transparency of the lower ipsilateral lung parenchyma *(arrowheads)*.

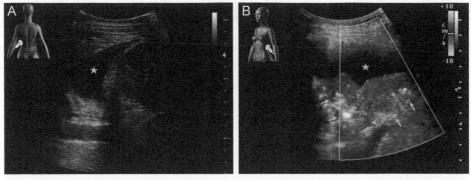

Fig. 17.3 Chest ultrasonography showing lesions in pulmonary embolism. (A) Anechoic pleural effusion *(star)*. (B) Peripheral lung consolidation *(arrows)* with vascular sign in color Doppler ultrasonography *(arrowhead)* and pleural anechoic effusion *(star)*.

Discussion Topic

Emergency room doctor

Most likely the patient has left pneumonia with parapneumonic pleural effusion.

Pulmonologist A

There are many signs compatible with infection. However, hemoptysis is rarely caused by pneumonia, unless it is necrotizing pneumonia or lung abscess. But why should it occur in a young woman without comorbidities or risk factors for complications?

Pulmonologist B

Moreover, the chest pain began before the fever.

Emergency room doctor

Do you think that it could be a pulmonary embolism?

Pulmonologist A

It's worth making an attempt to rule it out. Peripheral pulmonary consolidations are often seen on ultrasonography when embolic vascular occlusion causes necrosis of lung parenchyma.

Continued

Discussion Topic—cont'd

Pulmonologist B

Many, but not all, lesions appear as pleural-based and wedge-shaped parenchymal alterations at ultrasonography. Sometimes color Doppler imaging shows a congested thromboembolic vessel at the margin, called *vascular sign.* These findings support the diagnosis of pulmonary embolism.

Emergency room doctor

I believe we should also include blood and sputum cultures, as well as tests for tuberculosis in the diagnostic pathway

Clinical Course

It was determined that the patient was at moderate risk for pulmonary embolism, according to the Well's criteria. D-dimer was elevated (620 ng/mL, normal values < 250 ng/mL); thus the patient underwent computed tomography pulmonary angiography (CTPA), which showed filling defects caused by emboli in the left lower lobe segmental artery and the subsegmental branches supplying the anteromedial and lateral basal segments. CTPA also confirmed left pleural effusion and revealed irregular lung hyperdensity in the left lower lobe suggestive of pulmonary hemorrhage and infarction (Fig. 17.4).

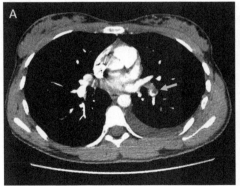
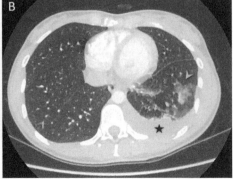

Fig. 17.4 Computer tomography pulmonary angiography (CTPA) image (A) showing a filling defect in a pulmonary arterial branch of the lower left lobe *(arrow)*. At the lung window level (B), a left pleural effusion *(star)* and consolidations in the left lower lobe *(arrowhead)* are evident.

Discussion Topic

Pulmonologist A

I didn't expect such extensive pulmonary embolism without respiratory failure and with only a slight increase in D-dimer.

Discussion Topic—cont'd

Pulmonologist B

It's not unusual for young individuals to maintain good oxygenation despite pulmonary embolism.

Internist

The increase in D-dimer is not so slight. Our hospital lab uses D-dimer units (DDU), which should be less than 250 ng/mL. So our patient has a value more than double the upper normal limit!

Other labs use fibrinogen equivalent units (FEU), which should be no higher than 500 ng/mL, or age multiplied by 10 in subjects older than 50 years of age.

Pulmonologist A

Can the contraceptive pill alone cause pulmonary embolism or, more broadly, venous thromboembolism (VTE)?

Internist

Probably no: it's better to investigate the patient for other possible risk factors and underlying thrombophilia.

Pulmonologist A

Which thrombophilia tests should be performed?

Internist

Because of this patient's age, a comprehensive assessment should include inherited and acquired conditions. Inherited thrombophilia states include gain-of-function mutations, such as those of factor V Leiden, and low levels of natural anticoagulants, as occurs in protein C or S deficiencies: these are less common but associated with a higher risk of VTE.

The most clinically relevant acquired hypercoagulable state is antiphospholipid syndrome, in which pathological antibodies may cause both venous and arterial thromboses.

Other conditions associated with increased thromboembolic risk are persistently elevated factor VIII and hyperhomocysteinemia. These can be both hereditary and acquired.

Pulmonologist B

Antiphospholipid antibodies include lupus anticoagulant (LAC), anticardiolipin antibodies, and anti-β_2-glycoprotein I antibodies, right?

Internist

Yes, you are correct! Remember that acute VTE and anticoagulant therapy may alter these test results and cause false-positive or false-negative findings. You should perform them at least 4 to 6 weeks after the acute event and after discontinuation of anticoagulant drugs. Moreover, diagnosis requires positivity of one or more of these three antibodies on two occasions more than 12 weeks apart.

Continued

Discussion Topic—cont'd

Pulmonologist A

Ventilation/perfusion V/Q lung scan could be useful to better evaluate the perfusion defect.

Pulmonologist B

It may be suitable when the diagnostic algorithm is inconclusive or CTPA cannot be performed because of allergy to iodine contrast medium or in the presence of chronic kidney disease. I believe it's not necessary for our patient at this moment because the presence of pulmonary embolism is already certain.

Pulmonologist A

The V/Q lung scan could be useful in the follow-up because it exposes the patient to less ionizing radiation compared with additional CTPA. Single-photon emission computed tomography (SPECT) or SPECT combined with low-dose CT (SPECT/CT) could be a valid alternative. There is increasing evidence that these have improved accuracy compared with planar V/Q scintigraphy.

Internist

I disagree about using imaging for follow-up. These methods expose the patients to radiation but don't guide treatment choices. So in my opinion, no further imaging is needed.

Pulmonologist B

Pulmonary infarcts can leave lung scars and pleural thickening. Imaging after clinical healing may be useful if suspected relapse occurs in the future.

Echocardiography showed normal size and function of the right atrium and ventricle, without any increase in arterial pulmonary pressure. Color Doppler ultrasonography excluded deep venous thrombosis (DVT) of lower limbs. Anticoagulant therapy was initiated with the subcutaneous injection of fondaparinux 5 mg once daily (which is the therapeutic dosage for people weighing < 50 kg). The patient experienced progressive clinical improvement and no longer had a fever or hemoptysis. The tuberculin skin test with 5 tuberculin units (TU) yielded a negative result. Blood and sputum cultures showed no growth. After a few days, the back pain occurred only during exertion or deep breathing, and pleural effusion decreased. No invasive procedure was performed.

Therapy and Further Indications at Discharge

The patient was discharged after 6 days of hospitalization. The oral contraceptive pill was discontinued. A direct oral anticoagulant (DOAC) was prescribed as home therapy (edoxaban, 30 mg once a day, which is the therapeutic dosage for people weighing < 60 kg).

The following outpatient follow-up was scheduled:

After 1 month: Thrombophilia screening (to be repeated in case of any positivity) and chest radiography

After 3 months: Single-photon emission computed tomography (SPECT) and pulmonary function tests

After 6 months: Echocardiography.

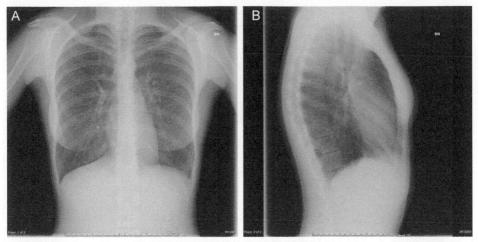

Fig. 17.5 Posteroanterior (A) and lateral (B) chest radiograph showing normal findings. The examination was performed 1 month after the acute pulmonary embolism.

Follow-Up and Outcomes

The patient experienced complete alleviation of pain within 2 weeks after discharge, and she no longer used pain relievers. No bleeding complications occurred. The patient resumed light physical activity, with good exercise tolerance. The chest ultrasonography and radiography results were normal (Fig. 17.5). Pulmonary function tests showed global volumes and lung diffusion capacity within normal limits. SPECT performed 3 months after the acute episode showed a large triangular fixation defect (lack of perfusion) of the radiopharmaceutical in the posterolateral region of the left lower lung lobe (Fig. 17.6).

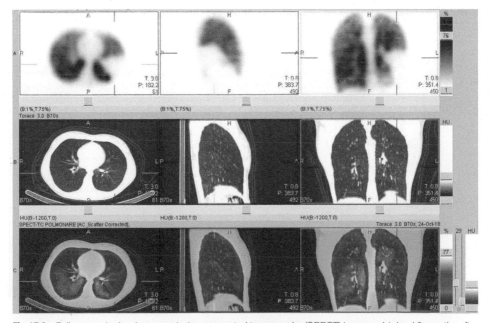

Fig. 17.6 Follow-up single-photon emission computed tomography (SPECT) images obtained 3 months after discharge). Despite normal computed tomography (CT) findings, a large triangular perfusion defect is evident in the posterolateral region of the lower left lung lobe.

An increase in factor VIII plasma activity level (214% or international units [IU]/dL, normal range 50–147% or IU/dL) was found at the first thrombophilia screening. However, this was not confirmed after further screening at 3 and 6 months (130% and 112%, respectively). The oral anticoagulant was discontinued after 6 months of treatment. No recurrence of pulmonary embolism occurred in the 2 years after the acute episode.

Discussion Topic

Pulmonologist A

I noticed that you stopped the anticoagulant after 6 months of therapy. Wasn't it better to continue it to reduce the risk of recurrence?

Internist

Given the temporal relationship between pulmonary embolism and contraceptive use, I believe that cessation of contraceptive use is sufficient to reduce the risk of recurrence.

Pulmonologist B

I agree. In a patient with a first episode and a major temporary risk factor, the risk is high only in the initial months after the acute episode, and anticoagulant can be discontinued after 3 or 6 months. The contraceptive pill is, however, only a minor temporary risk factor. According to the DASH (D-dimer, Age, Sex, Hormonal therapy) prediction score for recurrent venous thromboembolism (VTE), the patient's annual risk for VTE recurrence is 1% (Table 17.1).

Pulmonologist A

What role did the increase in factor VIII play?

Internist

It was increased only in one circumstance after hospitalization. A rise in factor VIII activity can be observed just after acute pulmonary embolism or during other inflammatory episodes. Only a persistently high value can be considered a risk factor for VTE.

Pulmonologist B

Exactly. Let's not forget that long-term anticoagulant treatment has a risk of causing major bleeding of 1% to 3% per year. It should be reserved for unprovoked or recurrent VTE.

Pulmonologist A

I agree with your proposal for therapy. However, beware that such a bleeding risk exists with use of vitamin K antagonists and is related to concomitant comorbid conditions. Direct oral anticoagulants have been shown to have a lower risk, and this is even lower in young patients.

TABLE 17.1 ■ DASH Prediction Score for Recurrent VTE and Relative Interpretation

DASH Item	Answer Choices	
D-dimer abnormal result	No (0)	Yes (2)
Age ≤ 50 years	No (0)	Yes (1)
Gender	Female (0)	Male (1)
Hormone use at VTE onset	Yes (−2)	No (0)

DASH	VTE Annual Recurrence Risk	Action After 3–6 Months
−2	1.80%	
−1	1%	Discontinue anticoagulation.
0	2.40%	
1	3.90%	
2	6.30%	
3	10.80%	Continue anticoagulation.
4	19.90%	

In patients receiving anticoagulation treatment after an unprovoked VTE event, anticoagulation can be discontinued after 3 to 6 months if the DASH score is 1 or less. In patients with scores greater than 2, the recommendation is to continue the therapy.

DASH, D-dimer, Age, Sex, Hormonal therapy; *VTE,* venous thromboembolism.

Focus On

Well's Criteria for Pulmonary Embolism: Three-Tier Model

Use of Well's Criteria for pulmonary embolism is one of the most common methods to estimate the probability of acute pulmonary embolism (PE).

The score is calculated as follows:
- Clinical signs and symptoms of deep venous thrombosis (DVT) = 3 points
- An alternative diagnosis is less likely than that of pulmonary embolism = 3 points
- Heart rate greater than 100/min = 1.5 points
- Immobilization for 3 or more consecutive days or surgery in the previous 4 weeks = 1.5 points
- Previous objectively diagnosed PE or DVT = 1.5 points
- Hemoptysis = 1 point
- Malignancy (with treatment in last 6 months or palliative treatment) = 1 point

If the patient is determined to be low risk (< 2 points) or moderate risk (score 2–6 points) for pulmonary embolism, D-dimer testing is recommended. If D-dimer level is normal, PE may be ruled out without further testing; if D-dimer is elevated, further imaging testing (e.g., computed tomography pulmonary angiography [CTPA] and/or ventilation/perfusion lung scan is warranted.

If it is determined that the patient is at high risk (score > 6 points), an imaging test, without measurement of D-dimer, is recommended.

Focus On

Lung Infarction With or Without Pulmonary Hemorrhage After Pulmonary Embolism

Acute pulmonary embolism (PE) may provoke pulmonary infarction with or without hemorrhage. Large emboli may cause acute cor pulmonale and sudden death without pathological changes in the lungs, whereas smaller emboli can lodge distally, causing lung damage and bleeding in the alveolar spaces. Pleuritic pain and/or hemoptysis are the most common clinical consequences of such events. The term *hemoptysis/pleuritic pain syndrome* (previously known as *pulmonary infarction syndrome*) is used for such presentation, which occurs in greater than 40% of all patients with PE, with pleuritic chest pain being more frequently observed than hemoptysis.

Pulmonary infarction is necrosis of a section of lung parenchyma, most often caused by thromboembolic disease. Lung infarction occurs infrequently because the lung is extensively vascularized by two systems (pulmonary and bronchial) with many mutual anastomoses. Moreover, the lungs also receive oxygen from inspired air.

The site of the occlusion, the rapidity of onset of embolism, and the compensation of arterial blood flow by other vessels may influence the occurrence of lung infarction.

The most common radiographic presentation of lung infarction is a wedge-shaped opacity with the base at the pleura.

It is important to note that pulmonary infarction and hemorrhage invariably occur in a subpleural location.

Predisposing factors for pulmonary infarction include low body mass index, active smoking, and age greater than 40 years.

Focus On

Pleural Effusion in Pulmonary Embolism

Pleural effusion occurs in approximately 30% to 50% of patients with pulmonary embolism (PE). Greater than 75% of patients with pleural effusions caused by PE have pleuritic chest pain. Therefore the presence of pleuritic chest pain in a patient with pleural effusion is highly suggestive of PE. At least half the patients younger than 40 years of age with pleural effusion and pleuritic chest pain have PE.

Pleuritic chest pain has been described as having a "stitch in the side" or a "stabbing" or "shooting" pain that may be exacerbated by deep inspiration, coughing, or sneezing. Pleural effusions caused by PE are generally small, ranging from just blunting of the costophrenic angle to less than one-third of the hemithorax in 90% of patients. They usually are exudates and, frequently, hemorrhagic. They can be loculated, especially if the diagnosis is delayed longer than 10 days after onset of symptoms. No specific treatment is usually required for these pleural effusions, and the presence of bloody pleural fluid is not a contraindication for the administration of anticoagulant therapy.

LEARNING POINTS

- Ultrasonography findings of pleural effusion and wedged-shaped lung consolidations with a vascular sign are highly suggestive of pulmonary embolism.
- Pulmonary embolism in young people may occur without respiratory failure.
- Pleural effusion, chest pain, and hemoptysis are suggestive of pulmonary embolism.
- Pulmonary infarction and hemorrhage occur at the periphery of the lung and may irritate the pleura, causing pain and pleural effusion.
- Thrombophilia testing is suggested in patients with unprovoked venous thromboembolism (VTE), recurrent VTE, VTE in unusual sites, VTE occurring at a young age, or a family history of VTE.
- High plasma level of factor VIII is a risk factor for isolated pulmonary embolism, but its value should be verified several months after an acute episode.

Further Reading

1. Bray TJP, Mortensen KH, Gopalan D. Multimodality imaging of pulmonary infarction. *Eur J Radiol.* 2014;83(12):2240–2254.
2. Baj M, Sorino C. Single photon emission computed tomography in the evaluation of lung diseases. In: Sorino C, ed. *Diagnostic Evaluation of the Respiratory System.* 1st ed. New Delhi, India: Jaypee Brothers Medical Publishers; 2017.
3. Squizzato A, Rancan E, Dentali F, et al. Diagnostic accuracy of lung ultrasound for pulmonary embolism: a systematic review and meta-analysis. *Thromb Haemost.* 2013;11:1269–1278.
4. Erkekol FO, Ulu A, Numanoglu N, Akar N. High plasma levels of factor VIII: an important risk factor for isolated pulmonary embolism. *Respirology.* 2006;11(1):70–74.
5. Findik S. Pleural effusion in pulmonary embolism. *Curr Opin Pulm Med.* 2012;18(4):347–354.
6. Nakashima MO, Rogers HJ. Hypercoagulable states: an algorithmic approach to laboratory testing and update on monitoring of direct oral anticoagulants. *Blood Res.* 2014;49:85–94.
7. Stein PD, Henry JW. Acute pulmonary embolism presenting as pulmonary hemorrhage/infarction syndrome in the elderly. *Am J Geriatr Cardiol.* 1998;7(3):36-42.
8. Stein PD, Beemath A, Matta F, et al. Clinical characteristics of patients with acute pulmonary embolism: data from PIOPED II. *Am J Med.* 2007;120(10):871–879.
9. Light RW. Pleural effusion in pulmonary embolism. *Semin Respir Crit Care Med.* 2010;31(6):716–722.
10. Garwood S, Strange C, Sahn SA. Massive hemoptysis. In: Parrillo JE, Dellinger RP, ed. *Critical Care Medicine. Principles of Diagnosis and Management in the Adults.* 3rd ed. St. Louis, MO: Elsevier; 2008.
11. Tosetto A, Iorio A, Marcucci M, et al. Predicting disease recurrence in patients with previous unprovoked venous thromboembolism: a proposed prediction score (DASH). *J Thromb Haemost.* 2012;10(6):1019–1025.
12. Wells PS, Anderson DR, Rodger M, et al. Excluding pulmonary embolism at the bedside without diagnostic imaging: management of patients with suspected pulmonary embolism presenting to the emergency department by using a simple clinical model and D-dimer. *Ann Intern Med.* 2001;135:98–107.
13. Righini M, Van Es J, Den Exter PL, et al. Age-adjusted D-dimer cutoff levels to rule out pulmonary embolism: the ADJUST-PE study [published correction appears in JAMA. 2014 Apr 23-30;311(16):1694]. *JAMA.* 2014;311:1117–1124.
14. Konstantinides SV, Torbicki A, Agnelli G, et al. Task Force for the Diagnosis and Management of Acute Pulmonary Embolism of the European Society of Cardiology (ESC). 2014 ESC guidelines on the diagnosis and management of acute pulmonary embolism. *Eur Heart J.* 2014;35:3033–3069.
15. van Es N, Kraaijpoel N, Klok FA, et al. The original and simplified Wells rules and age-adjusted D-dimer testing to rule out pulmonary embolism: an individual patient data meta-analysis. *J Thromb Haemost.* 2017;15:678–684.
16. Zhu R, Ma XC. Clinical value of ultrasonography in diagnosis of pulmonary embolism in critically ill patients. *J Transl Int Med.* 2017;5(4):200–204.
17. Mathis G, Blank W, Reissig A, et al. Thoracic ultrasound for diagnosing pulmonary embolism: a prospective multicenter study of 352 patients. *Chest.* 2005;128(3):1531–1538.
18. Comert SS, Caglayan B, Akturk U, et al. The role of thoracic ultrasonography in the diagnosis of pulmonary embolism. *Ann Thorac Med.* 2013;8(2):99–104.

CHAPTER 18

Bilateral Asymmetrical Pleural Effusion Due to Congestive Heart Failure

Claudio Sorino ■ Mario Tamburrini ■ David Feller-Kopman

History of Present Illness

An 80-year-old man presented to a cardiologist because he had worsening dyspnea and asthenia. Chest radiography showed right pleural effusion (Fig. 18.1). The cardiologist prescribed increased dosage of a loop diuretic (furosemide), an angiotensin-converting enzyme (ACE) inhibitor (enalapril), and an aldosterone receptor blocker (spironolactone). However, the patient became increasingly fatigued and confused. Arterial hypotension developed, and urine output decreased. Chest radiography showed an increase in the right pleural effusion, and blood tests revealed prerenal acute kidney injury. The patient was therefore admitted to the geriatric department.

Past Medical History

The patient was a retired office clerk, a former smoker (about 10 cigarettes a day for 25 years; he had quit 40 years before the current presentation). He had coronary artery disease (CAD), with residual diffuse myocardial hypokinesia and reduced left ventricular ejection fraction (LVEF: 25%). Two years earlier, a dual-chamber implantable cardioverter defibrillator

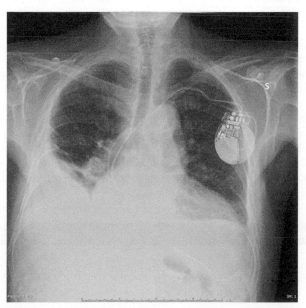

Fig. 18.1 Posteroanterior chest radiograph showing right pleural effusion.

(DR-ICD) was implanted. Three months before his current presentation, the patient had undergone right thoracentesis, and 1500 mL of transudative pleural fluid had been extracted. The patient also suffered from high blood pressure, type 2 diabetes mellitus, hypercholesterolemia, bilateral hearing loss, gallbladder stones, and central sleep apnea syndrome. He habitually used a bilevel positive airway pressure (BiPAP) device and oxygen therapy during the night. His home pharmacological therapy included acetylsalicylic acid 100 mg per day, omeprazole 20 mg per day, furosemide 125 mg two times daily, allopurinol 300 mg per day, metformin 500 mg two times daily, ursodeoxycholic acid 300 mg two times daily, enalapril 20 mg per day, and spironolactone 25 mg two times daily.

Physical Examination and Early Clinical Findings

At admission, the patient was afebrile, pale, confused, and complaining of breathlessness with minimal activity. Oxygen saturation (SpO_2) measured with pulse oximetry was 88% on room air. Arterial blood gas (ABG) analysis showed significant hypoxemia, with partial pressure of oxygen (PaO_2) of 53 mm Hg. Heart rate was 88 beats/min, respiratory rate was 20 breaths/min, and blood pressure was 90/50 mm Hg. On chest examination, breath sounds were absent in the lower right hemithorax, with dullness on percussion and decreased fremitus. Small symmetrical lower limb edema was also evident.

Blood tests showed high levels of serum creatinine (2.6 mg/dL), urea (102 mg/dL), and potassium (6.1 mEq/L). Total white blood cells (WBC) count was normal (7,220 cells/mm³) as were the inflammatory markers (C-reactive protein [CRP] < 10 mg/L). Hemoglobin was 11.2 g/dL, and platelet count was 120,000 cells/µL. Serum protein electrophoresis revealed only a slight reduction in total proteins (5.6 g/dL) and albumin (3.3 g/dL). Electrocardiography (ECG) showed sinus tachycardia, previously known left bundle branch block, left ventricular hypertrophy, prolonged corrected QT interval (QTc 490 ms).

Clinical Course

The patient received 40% oxygen via a Venturi mask, intravenous dopamine at intermediate rates of infusion (5 µg/kg/min), and oral sodium polystyrene sulfonate (15 mg every 6 hours). Enalapril and spironolactone were stopped. Administration of furosemide was changed to the intravenous route. Thoracic ultrasonography (Fig. 18.2) revealed a large area of right pleural effusion, with a flattened diaphragm, that was appreciable through four intercostal spaces and a small area of pleural effusion on the left. Additional signs of fluid overload were noted: both lungs showed vertical pulmonary artifacts (B-lines), and the inferior vena cava had increased in size and decreased in respiratory variability.

Chest computed tomography (CT) confirmed these findings and demonstrated absence of significant pulmonary parenchymal lesions, except for pulmonary atelectasis adjacent to the pleural effusion (Fig. 18.3).

In a few days, diuresis became adequate, and kidney function improved. However, the pleural effusion persisted, and the patient still needed supplemental oxygen at rest and had shortness of breath even on slight exertion.

Discussion Topic

Can you perform thoracentesis?

Geriatrician

Discussion Topic—cont'd

Pulmonologist

The evacuation of pleural fluid in heart failure has no role other than relief of symptoms. You should strengthen medical therapy.

Cardiologist

Medical therapy is already at the maximum!

Pulmonologist

If you believe that the dyspnea is caused by the pleural effusion, I am willing to do thoracentesis.

Cardiologist

Surely congestive heart failure (CHF) is the main cause of fatigue in the patient. However, if we allow his right lung to expand, I think that he can tolerate effort better. Maybe he could do without oxygen.

Geriatrician

And if the CHF was not the only cause of the pleural effusion? Our patient has fluid mainly on one side!

Pulmonologist

Pleural fluid was already analyzed a few months ago. It was a clear transudate. Moreover, no pulmonary parenchymal lesions were seen on the chest computed tomography (CT) scan.

Geriatrician

Could it be the onset of a primary tumor of the pleura?

Pulmonologist

I don't think so. However, given the patient's age and morbidity, more invasive diagnostic procedures are not recommended.

Right therapeutic thoracentesis was performed, and a large amount of fluid (1700 mL) was drained. The patient had no cough during the procedure and obtained subjective relief of dyspnea soon after. Pleural fluid analysis showed that it was still a transudate, with protein at 2.7 g/dL and lactate dehydrogenase (LDH) at 105 units/L. The search for malignant tumor cells on cytological

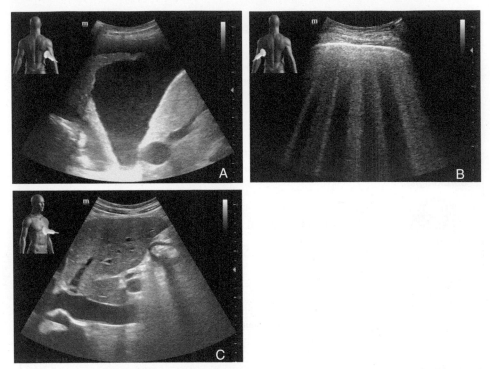

Fig. 18.2 Chest ultrasonography (convex probe) scans demonstrating large right pleural effusion (A); vertical pulmonary artefacts (B-lines) (B); and increased size of inferior vena cava (C).

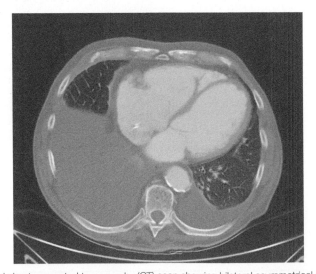

Fig. 18.3 Axial chest computed tomography (CT) scan showing bilateral asymmetrical pleural effusion.

examination yielded negative results. In the following days, oxygen saturation (SpO_2) increased to 92% at rest in room air. The patient was discharged, without a requirement for oxygen use during daylight hours.

Follow-Up and Outcomes

Four weeks after discharge, the patient was evaluated in the outpatient clinic. He was still fatigued and dyspneic with minimal effort. Blood pressure was low (100/60 mm Hg), but diuresis was sufficient, and serum creatinine was normal. Thoracic ultrasonography showed recurrence of the right pleural effusion, again appreciable through four intercostal spaces.

Discussion topic

Cardiologist

Pleural effusion relapsed again. However, I don't think the patient can benefit from a further increase in diuretic therapy. Blood pressure is low, and in such a circumstance, a prerenal acute kidney injury has already occurred.

Geriatrician

Could we perform another therapeutic thoracentesis?

Pulmonologist

We did it twice already. Did the patient get any relief?

Cardiologist

The patient says yes, but the improvement in his symptoms only lasted a few days.

Pulmonologist

We can propose insertion of an indwelling pleural catheter (IPC) to improve his quality of life.

Geriatrician

Can this promote pleurodesis?

Pulmonologist B

Yes, it can. However, in CHF, it occurs less frequently than in other conditions, such as malignancies or infections.
   Let me be clear: Actually, pleurodesis is not the purpose of the IPC, but rather alleviation of dyspnea.

Cardiologist

I agree. Our goal now is to ensure the best quality of life for the patient with end-stage heart disease.

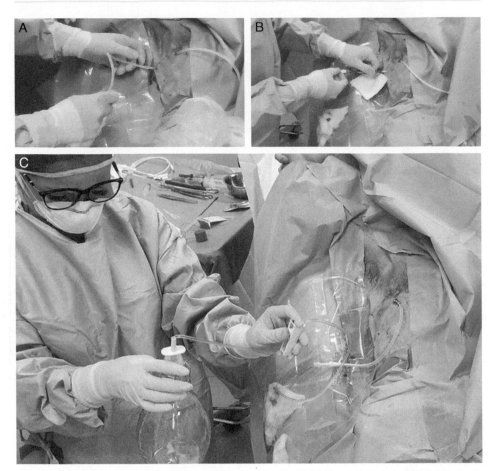

Fig. 18.4 Different phases of indwelling pleural catheter placement. (A) The catheter is tunneled subcutaneously between the two small skin incisions. (B) Chest tube insertion into the pleural cavity. (C) The indwelling pleural catheter (IPC) is connected to the vacuum drainage bottle.

The patient was made aware of the possible advantages and risks of placement of an indwelling pleural catheter (IPC). He accepted this treatment option, and the IPC was placed in the right chest (Fig. 18.4) as an outpatient procedure. The patient and his caregivers received education on its proper use and care. After immediate evacuation of 1500 mL of pleural fluid, the daily volume of the drainage gradually decreased. However, around 150 mL/day continued to be drained. No bleeding or infection occurred. Therefore the IPC was maintained. Heart failure continued to worsen, the patient developed progressive end-stage kidney disease, and died 2 months later.

Focus On

Pleural Effusions From Cardiovascular Diseases

Pleural effusion secondary to cardiovascular diseases is commonly encountered in clinical practice. It can be caused by congestive heart failure (CHF) or developed during pericardial diseases, after coronary artery bypass surgery, after heart transplantation, and in post–cardiac injury (Dressler) syndrome.

Focus On—cont'd

The incidence of CHF is high, and pleural effusion develops in over half the patients during their illness. Thus CHF is the most common cause of pleural effusions in developed countries. It results from elevated pulmonary capillary pressure, increased interstitial fluid in the lungs, and subsequent imbalance between the rate of pleural fluid formation and absorption.

The patient often has dyspnea out of proportion to the effusion size, orthopnea, or paroxysmal nocturnal dyspnea. Besides the signs of pleural effusion, physical examination usually reveals signs of right-sided heart failure, such as distended neck veins and peripheral edema, and signs of left-sided heart failure, such as rales and a third heart sound (S3 or ventricular gallop).

The diagnosis is usually suggested by the clinical picture of CHF. Chest radiography almost always reveals cardiomegaly and usually small- to medium-sized bilateral pleural effusions, which can be symmetrical or be larger on the right side. Routine diagnostic thoracentesis is not required unless the patient has unilateral pleural effusion or marked asymmetrical bilateral effusions, fever, leukocytosis, pleuritic chest pain, or absence of cardiomegaly. In these circumstances, alternative explanations should be investigated. The pleural fluid in a patient with CHF is typically a transudate. However, if the patient has been on diuretics, the ratio between pleural and blood values of proteins and lactate dehydrogenase (LDH) may be increased. In these settings, the serum–pleural fluid albumin gradient (serum albumin level minus pleural effusion albumin level) greater than 1.2 mg/dL or pleural fluid or serum N-terminal pro–brain natriuretic hormone (NT-proBNP) greater than 500 ng/mL is indicative of CHF.

Patients with CHF and pleural effusion should be treated with afterload reduction, diuretics, and inotropes, as needed.

Chest radiography and ultrasonography are used, alone or in combination, to monitor the effusion. Symptomatic patients with pleural effusion that does not resolve or that recurs despite maximal medical management may require evacuation of pleural fluid (therapeutic thoracentesis). In refractory cases, pleurodesis with the use of a sclerosing agent or the insertion of an indwelling catheter can be useful.

Focus On

Indwelling Pleural Catheters

Indwelling pleural catheters (IPCs) are palliative tools for the management of recurrent pleural effusions. Their role has expanded from second-line treatment for malignant effusions with trapped lung or failed pleurodesis to include primary therapy for several conditions. IPCs are effective in terms of both symptom control and costs, and can dramatically improve the patient's quality of life by offering the potential of a completely outpatient-driven solution.

The IPC is a multifenestrated chest drain made from a flexible silicone elastomer, with a small polyester cuff. The catheter is tunneled through a short section of subcutaneous tissue before the distal portion enters the pleural space, with the cuff then acting as a focal point for fibrous growth to allow the drain to remain in place. At the proximal (external) end is a one-way access valve designed to be attached to proprietary vacuum drainage bottles. The most common indications for inserting an indwelling catheter are malignant pleural effusions unsuitable for talc pleurodesis or recurrence after pleurodesis, trapped lung, and nonmalignant recurrent effusions, chylothorax, loculated effusions, and even empyema and hemothorax. Absolute contraindications include the inability of the patient, family, or health care services to manage the drain; uncorrected coagulopathy; pleural infection with ongoing sepsis; and cutaneous infection or significant malignant involvement over the proposed insertion site.

The IPC is introduced into the pleural space by using a modified Seldinger technique, with the catheter tunneled between two small skin incisions. These are usually created about 7 to 10 cm apart, allowing both easy access to the drain and sufficient length of the tunnel to reduce the risk of infection or dislodgement.

A typical initial IPC drainage frequency is three times per week, with subsequent adjustment based on volume drained and drainage-associated symptoms; normal drainage lasts around 15 min. A routine follow-up visit is generally scheduled for all patients 2 weeks after insertion. At this time, ultrasonography or chest radiography is performed, and symptoms, concerns, and complications are addressed.

The main advantages with IPC are patient satisfaction, decreased readmission rates, and reduced peri-intervention time in hospital. Complications associated with IPC are infrequent and include catheter-related pleural infections (cellulitis, empyema, tunnel infections), catheter tract metastasis, loculations, chest pain, and dislodgement or malfunction of the catheter (blockage, pericatheter leakage).

Focus On

IPCs in Nonmalignant Diseases

Pleural effusion is a common cause of breathlessness, cough, and chest pain. It may occur in patients with nonmalignant diseases and is associated with increased morbidity and mortality. The most common causes of nonmalignant pleural effusions (NMPEs) are congestive heart failure, hepatic hydrothorax (HH), chylothorax, renal failure, and lung transplantation. When pharmacological therapy fails, thoracentesis is often performed for symptom relief. It is common for the effusion to recur despite maximal medical therapy in these patient populations. In such circumstances, the placement of an indwelling pleural catheter (IPC) may be an effective and definitive therapeutic strategy, which is being increasingly used.

Although NMPEs are more common than malignant pleural effusions, evidence regarding the use of IPCs in NMPEs is more limited. Placement of an IPC results in immediate and sustained symptom relief. Moreover, it also potentially leads to pleurodesis without using sclerosing agents. This is a convenient advantage of IPC and occurs after approximately 6 weeks in nearly half the patients, more frequently in postinfectious effusions. How exactly the use of IPC leads to pleurodesis remains unclear; however, mechanical irritation causing local inflammation likely plays a role. As a consequence, pleurodesis is less common in older patients and those with cirrhosis and HH because they often have an altered inflammatory response.

Before proceeding with IPC, the underlying cause of the NMPE should be confirmed, and all providers, including potential heart and liver transplantation teams, should be included in the decision making. The primary goal of symptom control and satisfactory palliation without the need for subsequent procedures with IPCs can be achieved in greater than 80% of cases.

LEARNING POINTS

- Thoracentesis is not needed in congestive heart failure (CHF) unless pleural effusion is unilateral/asymmetrical or the patient has fever, leukocytosis, chest pain, or absence of cardiomegaly.
- Use of the indwelling pleural catheter (IPC) is a valid option for recurrent pleural effusion that occurs despite maximal therapy for nonmalignant diseases.
- The only aim of pleural drainage in CHF is symptom relief.

Further Reading

1. Chee A, Tremblay A. The use of tunneled pleural catheters in the treatment of pleural effusions. *Curr Opin Pulm Med.* 2011;17(4):237–241.
2. Chambers DM, Abaid B, Gauhar U. Indwelling pleural catheters for nonmalignant effusions: evidence-based answers to clinical concerns. *Am J Med Sci.* 2017;354(3):230–235.
3. Mullon J, Maldonado F. Use of tunneled indwelling pleural catheters for palliation of nonmalignant pleural effusions. *Chest.* 2011;140:996A.
4. Depew ZS, Iqbal S, Mullon JJ, et al. The role for tunneled indwelling pleural catheters in patients with persistent benign chylothorax. *Am J Med Sci.* 2013;346:349–352.
5. Thornton RH, Miller Z, Covey AM, et al. Tunneled pleural catheters for treatment of recurrent malignant pleural effusion following failed pleurodesis. *J Vasc Interv Radiol.* 2010;21:696–700.
6. Almeida FA, Bruno DS, Faiz S, Hinrichs B, Eapen GA, Bashoura L. Hemothorax treated with indwelling tunneled pleural catheter: are all hemothoraces the same. *J Bronchology Interv Pulmonol.* 2011;18:261–264.
7. Krishnan M, Cheriyath P, Wert Y, et al. The untapped potential of tunneled pleural catheters. *Ann Thorac Surg.* 2015;100:2055–2057.

8. Potechin R, Amjadi K, Srour N. Indwelling pleural catheters for pleural effusions associated with end-stage renal disease: a case series. *Ther Adv Respir Dis*. 2015;9:22–27.
9. Srour N, Potechin R, Amjadi K. Use of indwelling pleural catheters for cardiogenic pleural effusions. *Chest*. 2013;144:1603–1608.
10. Patil M, Dhillon SS, Attwood K, et al. Management of benign pleural effusions using indwelling pleural catheters: a systematic review and meta-analysis. *Chest*. 2017;151:626–635.
11. Mercer RM, Hassan M, Rahman NM. The role of pleurodesis in respiratory diseases. *Expert Rev Respir Med*. 2018;12:323–334.

CHAPTER 19

Posttraumatic Hemothorax and Pneumothorax in a Patient on Oral Anticoagulant

Claudio Sorino ■ Alessandro Squizzato ■ Francesco Inzirillo
■ David Feller-Kopman

History of Present Illness

A 58-year-old Caucasian man was taken to the emergency room (ER) after a motorcycle accident (collision with a car). The patient had thoracic and head trauma.

Past Medical History

The patient had been suffering from paroxysmal atrial fibrillation for about 8 years and was regularly taking anticoagulant therapy for stroke prevention. One year earlier, vitamin K antagonist (warfarin, dose adjusted for a target international normalized ratio [INR] of 2–3) was replaced with a direct oral anticoagulant (dabigatran 150 mg two times daily). The patient had been using a nocturnal continuous positive airway pressure (CPAP) device for 5 years for obstructive sleep apnea syndrome (OSAS).

Physical Examination and Early Clinical Findings

At the ER, the patient was found to be alert and had pain in his right hemithorax. The first measurement of oxygen saturation showed very low values (SpO_2 78%) and the administration of oxygen 15 L/min via a face mask with reservoir (fraction of inspired oxygen [FiO_2] approximately 90%) was needed to obtain SpO_2 of 94% or greater. Breaths were frequent (around 40/min) and shallow. The patient had no signs of subcutaneous emphysema in the neck or chest. Breath sounds were reduced at the lower right pulmonary field.

Blood pressure was 105/70 mm Hg. Hemoglobin was 11.2 g/dL. Coagulation tests revealed an increase in prothrombin time (PT: 16 seconds; normal range 11.0–13.0 seconds), INR was 1.58 (normal values < 1.1), and activated partial thromboplastin time (aPTT) was 50 seconds (normal range 25–35 seconds). Leukocytes and inflammatory indices were just above the normal limits (white blood cell [WBC] count 11,900 cells/μL; C-reactive protein [CRP] 12 mg/L). The patient had an occipital scalp laceration, which was promptly closed with surgical staples.

The patient underwent total-body computed tomography (CT), which identified multiple bilateral rib fractures. On the right side, some ribs were broken in several parts, and a few bone fragments had reached the pleural cavity. Right pleural effusion suggestive of hemothorax (maximum thickness 27 mm) and thin right pneumothorax (maximum thickness 7 mm) were evident, as well as large hyperdensity in the right upper lobe, resulting from pulmonary contusion, and hyperdensity in the right lower lobe in contiguity with the pleural effusion, resulting from partial atelectasis (Figs. 19.1 and 19.2). The patient also had a spinous process fracture of the T2 vertebra, and bilateral slightly displaced sacral ala fractures at the level of S1–S3, without spinal cord injury. The findings from brain and abdomen CT were unremarkable.

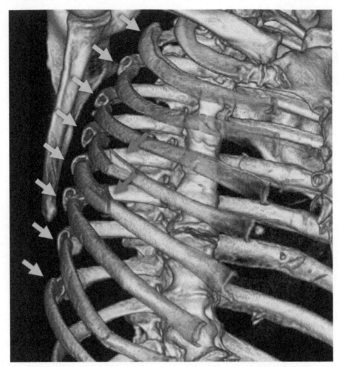

Fig. 19.1 Three-dimensional reconstruction of the chest computed tomography (CT) scan, showing multiple rib fractures *(yellow arrows)* with bone fragments displaced toward the pleural cavity *(blue arrows)*.

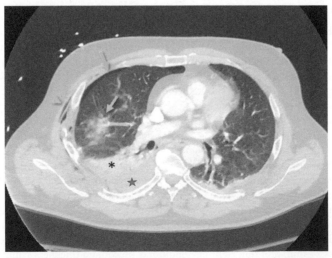

Fig. 19.2 Axial chest computed tomography (CT) scan showing right pleural effusion *(blue star)*, small right pneumothorax *(green arrow)*, small subcutaneous emphysema *(yellow arrowhead)*, hyperdensity in the right upper lobe caused by pulmonary contusion *(yellow arrow)*, and right lower lobe hyperdensity in contiguity with the pleural effusion *(black asterisk)*.

Clinical Course

Opioid analgesics were administered (intravenous morphine 0.1 mg/kg during ambulance transport, followed by intravenous fentanyl 100 μg). The patient underwent endotracheal intubation and received invasive mechanical ventilation and then was admitted to the intensive care unit (ICU).

Discussion Topic

Intensivist

The extent of pleural effusion appears mild, and pneumothorax is minimal. Should we wait and see?

Pulmonologist A

I think it's not a good idea. The patient is likely to have had pleural bleeding. Most pleural effusions occurring after chest trauma are hemothorax.

Pulmonologist B

It's important to figure out if this is the case, because bleeding may continue and cause hypovolemic shock. In a patient with traumatic hemothorax, 3 to 4 liters of blood may rapidly accumulate in the pleural cavity!

Pulmonologist A

If there is blood inside the pleural cavity, it should be removed, even if the bleeding has stopped. Undrained hemothorax may subsequently evolve into fibrothorax.

Intensivist

You are right! It would be better to place a pleural drain. There is also a risk that the pneumothorax will get worse in the next few hours. A chest tube could prevent tension pneumothorax.

Pulmonologist B

Positioning a pleural drain will not be easy because of the multiple displaced rib fractures. I suggest using a small-bore chest tube and being very careful.

Pulmonologist A

Moreover, the patient is on anticoagulant therapy. He took the last dose of dabigatran this morning.

Intensivist

We have idarucizumab, which is a specific antidote to reverse the anticoagulant effect of dabigatran. Do you think it's appropriate to use it here?

Continued

Discussion Topic—cont'd

Pulmonologist A

The hemoglobin level is a bit low, and we have no previous values. We don't know how much the patient has bled and if he's still bleeding.

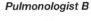

Pulmonologist B

The patient doesn't have frank hypotension, and hemoglobin values are far above the level requiring blood transfusion. Reversal agents for direct oral anticoagulants should be reserved for life-threatening bleeding.

They are also indicated before urgent surgery, but I think that they are not needed before placing a small-bore chest tube.

Intensivist

We can administrate prothrombin complex concentrate (PCC). This will allow for replacing coagulation factors and reducing the risk of further bleeding. PCC acts quickly, and you can perform the procedure after only 15 minutes.

Because the patient was deeply sedated and intubated, his wife gave the consent for thoracic drainage. Prothrombin complex concentrate (PCC) was administrated to obtain rapid replacement of coagulation factors. Under ultrasound guidance, the thoracic surgeon performed an exploratory puncture at the seventh right intercostal space along the middle axillary line. He used a syringe previously filled with anesthetic (lidocaine 20 mg/mL, 1 ampule of 10 mL corresponding to 200 mg). Dark blood came out of the pleural cavity. A subsequent small incision was made with the tip of the scalpel, and a small-bore pleural drain (12-French [Fr]) was placed. This was secured to the skin with a 2-0 silk suture and connected to an underwater seal drainage system. About 300 mL of dark blood was evacuated in a few minutes, and 200 mL of bloody fluid came out in the next 12 hours. Minor transient air leaks were observed as well. Chest radiography confirmed good drain positioning and showed reduction of pleural effusion.

Unfortunately, after a further 24 hours later, sudden worsening of the oxygen parameters was observed. The movements of the right hemithorax were extremely reduced, and breath sounds on this side were almost absent. Repeat chest CT revealed large right pneumothorax with slight contralateral displacement of the mediastinal structures (Fig. 19.3).

The thoracic surgeon then urgently placed a chest drain in the fourth right intercostal space, along the anterior axillary line (Fig. 19.4). Because adequate time had passed from suspension of the anticoagulant and because the hemoglobin level was stable, a large-bore chest tube (28-Fr) was used. It was secured to the skin with a 0 silk suture and connected to a three-chamber drainage system (Fig. 19.5). There was abundant air leakage, which persisted for several days, manifesting as continuous bubbling. The lower pleural drain was found to be blocked by clots and was therefore removed.

Discussion Topic

Intensivist

Air leak from the pleural drain is still visible. Would it be useful to apply suction?

Discussion Topic—cont'd

Pulmonologist A

I'm afraid not. Evidently one of the broken ribs pierced the lung, and the laceration is not yet repaired.

Pulmonologist B

Video-assisted thoracoscopic surgery (VATS) or thoracotomy may be indicated in case of prolonged air leakage.

Pulmonologist A

Although we assess bubbling three times a day, it's difficult to estimate whether the rate of daily air leakage is unchanged. We could replace the analog drainage system with a digital one.

Intensivist

What advantages would it have over the analog system?

Pulmonologist B

With a traditional system, you can see the air leak only during the medical visit. Electronic systems with continuous digital monitoring of air leakage provide a more precise balance of actual air leakage and provide a graphical display of its trend over time.

Intensivist

So, if air leakage reduces progressively, you could hypothesize that it will stop soon, thus avoiding surgery!

Pulmonologist B

In my opinion, the main real advantage of using digital devices is the higher interobserver agreement on when to remove the chest tube.

Pulmonologist A

Another advantage is the monitoring and storing of pleural pressure records. These are useful to predict the occurrence of prolonged air leak. Also, pleural pressure records may help differentiate active air leakage from a pleural space effect.

Pulmonologist B

The same can be obtained by using conventional systems, which cost less. You only need trained staff!

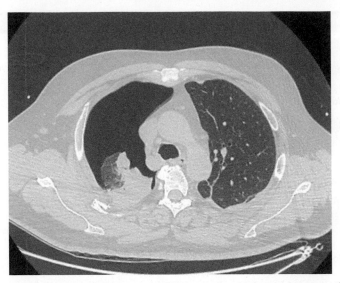

Fig. 19.3 Axial chest computed tomography (CT) scan showing large right pneumothorax.

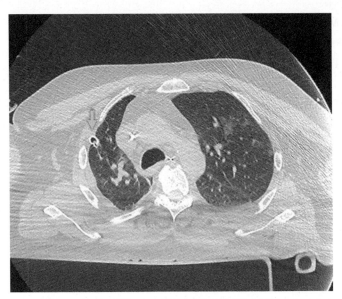

Fig. 19.4 Chest computed tomography (CT) scan obtained after insertion of the second pleural drain. Good expansion of the right lung was obtained. The chest tube is visible in the subpleural area *(yellow arrow)*.

The analogic drainage system was changed with a digital one. After finding that the hemoglobin level was stable, low-molecular-weight heparin (LMWH) was started on a prophylactic dosage for prevention of venous thromboembolism (VTE) (subcutaneous enoxaparin 4000 units/day), given the immobilization of the patient.

During the patient's stay in the ICU, significant retention of airway secretions interfered with ventilation and impaired gas exchange. Standard suctioning failed to clear the secretions;

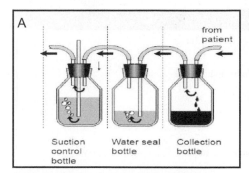

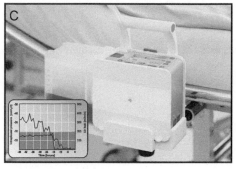

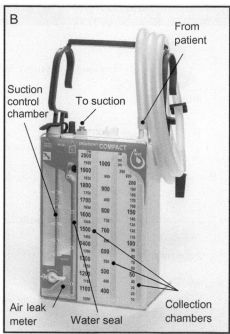

Fig. 19.5 Examples of drainage systems. (A) Schematization of a three-bottle system. The first chamber is for fluid collection, and the second contains a water seal and allows air removal. As the two are separate, fluid drainage does not adversely affect the pressure gradient for the evacuation of air from the pleural space. The third chamber allows for applying suction. (B) A modern analog chest drainage unit with three integrated chambers. (C) A digital system with relevant display showing the trends in air and fluid leakage. Used with the permission of REDAX.

thus toilet bronchoscopy was performed. Medical therapy included a broad-spectrum antibiotic (intravenous piperacillin/tazobactam 4/0.5 g three times daily), and a mucolytic/antioxidant agent (intravenous N-acetylcysteine 300 mg two times daily). After 8 days, the patient was extubated and received noninvasive ventilation alternating with periods of spontaneous breathing supported by oxygen supplement.

Bubbling from the chest tube became intermittent, and the digital drainage system showed progressive reduction in air leakage.

Discussion Topic

Intensivist

The patient's clinical condition has improved. Inflammatory indices are low. Can we stop the antibiotic therapy, or is it preferable to maintain it because the chest tube is still in place?

Pulmonologist A

Prophylactic antibiotics after a chest tube insertion do not reduce the incidence of empyema or pneumonia. So I believe it's not necessary to continue it.

Continued

Discussion Topic—cont'd

Intensivist

How long should such a drain be maintained?

Pulmonologist B

It should stay inserted until bubbling stops.

Intensivist

There has been no active air leakage for 24 hours. So could we remove the intercostal tube?

Pulmonologist A

It is preferable to clamp the drain and obtain a chest radiograph. If this doesn't show reaccumulation of air in the pleural cavity, we can remove the drain.

The patient was transferred to the pulmonology department. He resumed oral intake, and antibiotic therapy was stopped. No further air leakage was observed, and chest ultrasonography showed no increase of the right pleural effusion, but it showed the presence of two lung points localized in the insertion site of the pleural drain. The drain was removed 16 days after its placement.

The improvement in gas exchange allowed cessation of oxygen supplementation. Blood gas analysis, with the patient breathing ambient air, showed pH 7.41, partial pressure of oxygen (PaO_2) 78 mm Hg, and partial pressure of carbon dioxide ($PaCO_2$) 41.6 mm Hg.

The white blood cell (WBC) count and inflammatory indices normalized.

The bladder catheter was removed, and the patient resumed spontaneous urination, with no significant postvoid residual urine (approximately 30 mL).

Recommended Therapy and Further Indications at Discharge

Chest CT performed after removal of the second drain showed right-sided residual small hydropneumothorax (Fig. 19.6). The patient was discharged home with instructions to continue resting until the scheduled pneumological and orthopedic follow-up assessments.

Follow-Up and Outcomes

The patient visited the outpatient clinic 4 weeks after discharge. He remained afebrile and had no breathlessness at rest. He occasionally experienced mild right chest pain, which was well controlled with paracetamol taken as needed. The patient embarked on a rehabilitation program, and

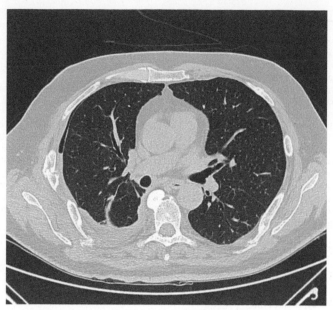

Fig. 19.6 Chest computed tomography (CT) scan obtained after removal of the second chest tube. Right residual small hydropneumothorax is evident.

after 2 months, he started walking with the help of crutches. Progressive leg loading was allowed, and after another month, crutches were no longer needed, and enoxaparin was stopped.

Eight months after discharge, the patient had regained autonomy in performing activities of daily life. Chest imaging revealed almost normal lung parenchymal findings, and no alterations were found in the pulmonary function test results.

Focus On

Hemorrhagic Pleural Effusions and Hemothorax

Hemothorax is the presence of blood in the pleural space. It is usually a consequence of chest trauma. Penetrating injuries of the lungs, heart, great vessels, diaphragm, or chest wall are obvious causes of hemothorax. In nonpenetrating chest injuries, the intercostal vessel or the internal mammary arteries are the most common sources of bleeding because they can be lacerated by a fractured rib.

Much less frequently, hemothorax is the complication of specific diseases—iatrogenic or spontaneous.

While an injury to the major arterial or venous structures of the thorax or of the heart itself may cause massive hemorrhage, hemothorax resulting from injuries to the pulmonary parenchyma is usually self-limiting because the pulmonary vascular pressure is low. Furthermore, it is often associated with pneumothorax.

The causes of spontaneous hemothorax include malignancies with pleural involvement, anticoagulant medications, hematological disorders (hemophilia), vascular ruptures (aortic dissection, arteriovenous malformations), endometriosis, pulmonary infarctions, and pleural adhesions (in association with pneumothorax).

The bloody appearance of pleural fluid is a frequent finding during thoracentesis. A pleural fluid hematocrit equal to or greater than 50% of the peripheral blood hematocrit usually confirms the diagnosis of hemothorax.

Chest ultrasonography has higher sensitivity and specificity compared with chest radiography in the diagnosis of hemothorax. On ultrasonography, hemothorax appears as an anechoic (black) or

Continued

Focus On—cont'd

echo-poor area of effusion, which occasionally contains heterogeneous echoes from clotted blood, debris, or portions of lacerated lung tissue.

High attenuation of pleural fluid on chest computed tomography (CT) (Hounsfield unit [HU] 35–70) aids in the diagnosis of hemothorax.

The initial treatment for hemothorax is tube thoracostomy. This is contraindicated when significant pleural adhesions are known to be present because their blunt division may cause lung laceration and additional bleeding.

Based on the initial volume output, the next step may be either urgent thoracotomy or observation. If the source of bleeding is the pulmonary parenchyma, hemostasis is usually achieved by complete expansion of the lung because the pulmonary circulation is a low-pressure circuit. Bleeding from lacerated intercostal or internal mammary arteries is likely to persist and may require urgent surgery for definitive hemostasis.

Video-assisted thoracoscopic surgery (VATS) permits direct removal of clots and precise placement of a chest tube. Open thoracotomy may be required if massive hemothorax or persistent bleeding is present. Inadequate hemothorax evacuation may be complicated by empyema or become organized and evolve to fibrothorax.

Focus On

Chest Drainage Systems

A chest drainage unit (CDU) is a sterile, disposable system designed to remove air and fluid from the pleural space, prevent their return, and restore negative pressure in the pleural cavity, thus promoting lung re-expansion.

A CDU consists of one or more chambers that collect fluid and a flexible tube, which is attached to the catheter exiting the pleural cavity. The CDU must be positioned below the level of the chest tube insertion to allow fluid to drain by gravity.

The thoracic drainage devices have evolved considerably since their introduction. There are several single or multiple collection chamber systems (Fig. 19.5).

The one-bottle system (also known as the *Bülau drain*) has a single unit with an underwater seal. A rigid straw, connected to the chest tube, enters the bottle and is immersed in normal saline solution so that its tip is located 2 cm below the surface of the saline. An opening with a one-way valve (vent) allows the system to be depressurized.

A two-bottle system has a first bottle (closer to the patient) for fluid collection, and a second bottle that contains the water seal and allows air removal. The two-bottle system is preferred over the one-bottle system when large quantities of pleural liquid have to be drained. As the two bottles are separate, fluid drainage does not adversely affect the pressure gradient for evacuation of air from the pleural space.

In three-bottle systems, a third bottle is added (suction control chamber) and is useful if suction is required.

Traditional CDUs regulate the amount of suction by the height of a column of water in the suction control chamber. Suction pressure up to –20 centimeters of water (cm H_2O) is commonly recommended.

All these chambers are currently integrated into modern, multifunctional, easy-to-manage boxes.

Advanced digital CDUs (smart drainage systems) offer digital flow recordings with an inbuilt alarm system. They facilitate accurate chest tube management by monitoring fluid and air leakage and pleural pressure. Data can be reviewed in a graphic format. Digital CDUs can be attached to a battery-powered smart suction device. This may afford early mobilization of the patient.

Focus On

Antidotes for the Reversal of Anticoagulants

Urgent complete reversal of the anticoagulant effect of vitamin K antagonists (VKAs) and direct oral anticoagulants (DOACs) is necessary in case of major or life-threatening bleeding, trauma, emergency surgery, or invasive procedures.

Focus On—cont'd

Patients with major or life-threatening VKA-associated bleeding should be promptly treated with prothrombin complex concentrate (PCC), at doses tailored on the basis of the international normalized ratio (INR) value, in addition to intravenous vitamin K. Fresh frozen plasma (FFP) should be used as first-line agent in case PCC is not immediately available.

Specific reversal antidotes for DOACs are now available (idarucizumab for dabigatran and andexanet alpha for factor Xa inhibitors). Idarucizumab is administered intravenously as two consecutive rapid boluses of 2.5 g, no more than 15 minutes apart. Andexanet alpha is administered as a bolus over 15 to 30 minutes, followed by a 2-hour infusion. The dose is dependent on the type of drug and time since the last intake. PCC can be considered for patients with life-threatening bleeding as part of factor Xa inhibitor therapy if immediate hemostatic support is required, especially in situations where a specific reversal agent is not available.

It should be noted that reversal agents may be beneficial only when their administration is integrated with a multimodal approach to bleeding, including the following:

- Withdrawal of the anticoagulant drug till local hemostasis is safe
- Blood tests to check for hemoglobin level, platelet count, renal and liver functions, coagulation parameters (prothrombin time [PT], activated partial thromboplastin time [aPTT]), and DOAC plasma level
- Red blood cell transfusion, platelet and/or administration of FFP and eventually tranexamic acid
- Management of any additional bleeding risk factors, such as uncontrolled hypertension, excessive alcohol intake, antithrombotic therapies (in particular, antiplatelet drugs), nonsteroidal antiinflammatory drugs, and glucocorticoids.

LEARNING POINTS

- Bloody pleural fluid with hematocrit ≥ 50% of the peripheral blood is termed *hemothorax*.
- In most cases, pleural effusion occurring after chest trauma is hemothorax.
- Digital drainage systems allow for precise monitoring of air leakage and may help determine when to remove a chest tube.
- PCC allows for rapid replacement of coagulation factors before initiation of invasive procedures.

Further Reading

1. Moia M, Squizzato A. Reversal agents for oral anticoagulant-associated major or life-threatening bleeding. *Intern Emerg Med.* 2019;14(8):1233–1239.
2. Novoa NM, Jiménez MF, Varela G. When to remove a chest tube. *Thorac Surg Clin.* 2017;27(1):41–46.
3. Lee YY, Hsu PK, Huang CS, Wu YC, Hsu HS. Complications after chest tube removal and reinterventions in patients with digital drainage systems. *J Clin Med.* 2019;8(12):2092.
4. Porcel JM. Chest tube drainage of the pleural space: a concise review for pulmonologists. *Tuberc Respir Dis (Seoul).* 2018;81(2):106–115.
5. Zisis C, Tsirgogianni K, Lazaridis G, et al. Chest drainage systems in use. *Ann Transl Med.* 2015;3(3):43.
6. Novoa NM, Fuentes MG. Digital chest drainage vs. water seal chest drainage in the robotic era. *J Thorac Dis.* 2020;12(6):3004–3006.
7. Bowman JA, Utter GH. Electronic chest tube drainage devices and low suction following video-assisted thoracoscopic pulmonary lobectomy. *J Thorac Dis.* 2019;11(5):1738–1741.

Pneumothorax After Transthoracic Needle Biopsy of the Lung

Claudio Sorino ■ Cecilia Sampietro ■ Angelo Calati ■ Giuseppe Pepe

History of Present Illness

A 79-year-old man presented to the outpatient pulmonary clinic with upper right opacity that was demonstrated on chest radiography, which had been performed during follow-up for high-grade papillary urothelial carcinoma.

A subsequent chest computed tomography (CT) revealed pulmonary hyperdensity in the right upper lobe apical segment. The hyperdensity was located in the anterior subpleural area and showed necrotic–colliquative features. A subsequent ^{18}F-fluorodeoxyglucose (FDG) positron emission tomography/computed tomography (PET/CT) showed that the pulmonary lesion had high glucose metabolism with maximum standardized uptake value (SUV_{max}) of 6.8 (Fig. 20.1). Other small hyperdense lung lesions were evident, with negligible FDG uptake.

Past Medical History

The patient was a smoker (about 10 cigarettes/day). Eleven years earlier, he had undergone lower left lobectomy for lung cancer (adenocarcinoma, G3 pT2 pN0 M0) and subsequent adjuvant chemotherapy with cisplatin plus vinorelbine (three cycles; negative long-term follow-up).

Eight years after lobectomy, the patient had undergone transurethral resection of bladder tumor (TURBT) and subsequent intravesical instillations with bacillus Calmette-Guérin (BCG) for high-grade papillary urothelial carcinoma.

The patient suffered from arterial hypertension, chronic gastritis, hypercholesterolemia, and prostatic hypertrophy. He also had undergone total thyroidectomy for Graves' disease and right total hip replacement for osteoarthritis, and he had recurrent venous thrombosis and bilateral pulmonary embolism. His usual therapy included levothyroxine, atenolol, amlodipine, esomeprazole, warfarin, atorvastatin, and tamsulosin.

Physical Examination and Early Clinical Findings

During pulmonary evaluation, the patient was alert, cooperative, fully active, and able to carry on normal activity, with breathlessness experienced only after moderate or intense effort. Despite his multiple pathologies, his performance status (PS) was 90%, according to the Karnofsky scale, corresponding to an Eastern Clinical Oncology Group PS (ECOG PS) score of 0. The patient was 177 cm tall and weighed 84 kg. Oxygen saturation (SpO_2) was 95% while breathing ambient air, and heart rate was 75 beats/min at rest. The patient had no pallor, cyanosis, or peripheral edemas. Chest examination showed only a slight diffuse reduction of breath sounds. Skin scarring resulting from surgery on the left hemithorax was visible. The abdomen was globular, with no obvious masses. Blood test results were within normal limits, except for the international normalized ratio (INR), which was 2.8 because of the use of warfarin.

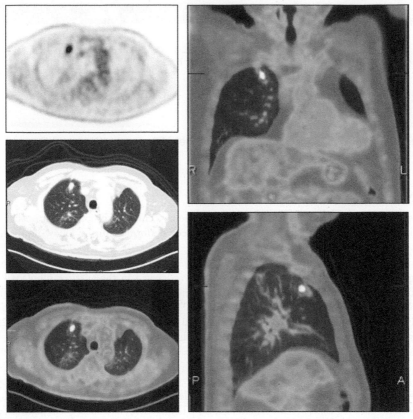

Fig. 20.1 Positron emission tomography/computed tomography (PET/CT) scan showing radiopharmaceutical hyperaccumulation in the anterior nodule of the right upper lung. The small hyperdense lesions in the posterior area had negligible fluorodeoxyglucose (FDG) uptake.

Discussion Topic

Radiologist

The pulmonary nodule in the right upper lobe could be metastasis of bladder cancer.

Pulmonologist

Yes, it can be, just as it can be primary lung cancer.

Oncologist

What is the probability that bronchoscopy will provide the diagnosis?

Discussion Topic—cont'd

Pulmonologist

Rather poor, because of the peripheral position of the lesion. Some bronchoscopic techniques, such as fluoroscopic guidance, radial endobronchial ultrasonography, and electromagnetic navigation, may help with biopsy of such lesions. The sensitivity of these techniques is 50% to 70%. The highest diagnostic yield is obtained when the operator is an expert, the nodule is greater than 3 cm in size, and computed tomography (CT) reveals a bronchus sign.

Radiologist

We could perform transthoracic needle aspiration (TTNA) or biopsy (TTNB).

Oncologist

What are the main differences between the two procedures?

Radiologist

With biopsy, more tissue is obtained, and its sensitivity is greater; thus it is my favorite choice. However, the risk of complications, such as pneumothorax, is also greater.

Oncologist

It can be a good choice. We have to stop warfarin and wait for the international normalized ratio (INR) to drop to 1.4 or less.

Clinical Course

Three days after discontinuation of warfarin, the INR was 1.34, and platelet count was normal. The patient was admitted to the oncology department and underwent CT-guided transthoracic needle biopsy (TTNB). At the end of the procedure, small right pneumothorax was evident (Fig. 20.2); therefore the patient was kept at rest. However, in the subsequent hours, he developed severe dyspnea, together with a slight reduction in SpO_2 (93%) and an increase in heart rate (90 beats/min). Subsequent chest radiography showed extension of the right pneumothorax, with partial collapse of the lung and contralateral displacement of the mediastinal structures (Fig. 20.3).

Discussion Topic

Pulmonologist

Do you believe that the lung can only expand with rest?

Continued

Thoracic surgeon

It is not excluded. However, the lung may collapse completely or the pneumothorax may further worsen and become hypertensive.

Pulmonologist

If a tension pneumothorax occurs in the night, urgent action would be needed. I would prefer not to take risks. I suggest placing a chest tube.

Thoracic surgeon

I agree. A small-bore chest tube will be enough!

Placement of a small-bore chest tube was proposed. After obtaining written consent from the patient, the thoracic surgeon injected a local anesthetic into the fifth right intercostal space, along the midaxillary line. When the needle reached the pleural space, air bubbles were evident in the syringe used for anesthesia. A 12-French (Fr) chest drain was then placed in this site and connected to a three-chamber drainage system (Fig. 20.4). Subsequent chest radiography showed good

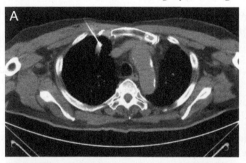

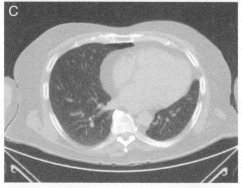

Fig. 20.2 Computed tomography (CT)–guided transthoracic needle biopsy of the upper right lung lesion. (A) Mediastinal window. (B) Parenchymal window. A subsequent small pneumothorax is evident (C).

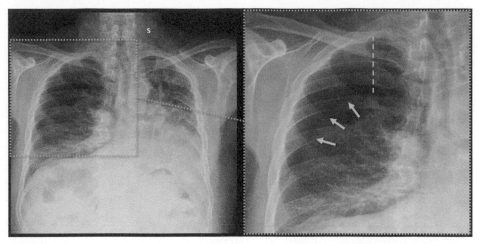

Fig. 20.3 Posteroanterior chest radiographs showing large right pneumothorax with a contralateral mediastinal shift. In the enlargement on the right, the yellow dotted line indicates the vertical thickness of pneumothorax. The arrows indicate the upper and lateral edge of the lung.

expansion of the right lung (Fig. 20.5). Given the patient's history of recurrent venous thromboembolism (VTE), and the probable presence of malignancy, administration of anticoagulant therapy was resumed 12 hours after chest tube placement.

The physicians chose to use subcutaneous enoxaparin (6000 units two times daily) because of its short half-life, which offered an advantage in case of bleeding or further invasive procedures.

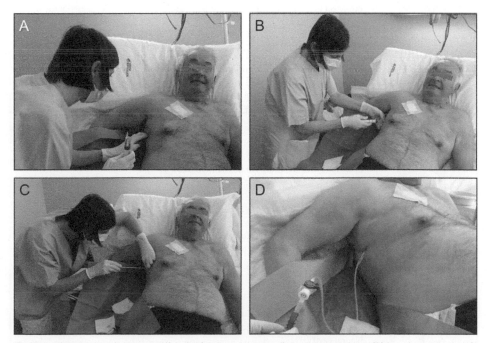

Fig. 20.4 Chest tube placement. (A) Individuation of the needle insertion position. (B) Local anesthesia. (C) Insertion of the catheter with needle and stylet into the pleural space. (D) The catheter has been placed and connected to the drainage system, and the needle has been removed.

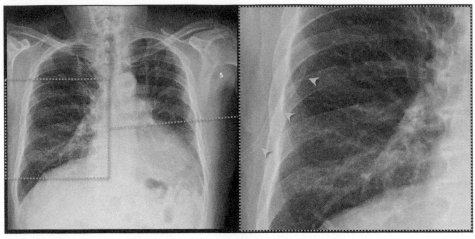

Fig. 20.5   Posteroanterior chest radiograph obtained after drainage *(enlargement on the right)*. The right lung has expanded, and the pneumothorax is no longer recognizable. The small-bore chest tube, crossing the chest wall, is barely visible *(yellow arrowheads)*.

Discussion Topic

Pulmonologist

Why did you place the chest tube sideways?

Thoracic surgeon

This is my preferred position. Here the needle does not have to cross a thick muscle layer, and the risk of damaging structures is minimal. This is why the axillary region is called the *safety triangle*. Furthermore, it is often more comfortable for the patient.

Oncologist

How long will the drainage be maintained?

Thoracic surgeon

Hard to say right now. Before removing the chest tube, we should verify that the lung is fully expanded and there is no more air leakage for at least 24 or 48 hours.

Pulmonologist

Maybe we should wait for the histological examination results. If further invasive diagnostic attempts are required, we could do them with the tube still in the pleural cavity.

Three days after chest tube placement, no further air leakage was evident. The patient was eupneic, and breath sounds were present bilaterally. After a further 2 days of observation, chest radiography showed a well-expanded right lung, and no lung point was evident on chest ultra-sonography. The histology of lung biopsy was lepidic-predominant adenocarcinoma (LPA) of the lung. No mutation of the epidermal growth factor receptor *(EGFR)* gene or rearrangements of the anaplastic lymphoma kinase *(ALK)* and reactive oxygen species 1 *(ROS1)* genes were found. The tumor cells had low programmed death ligand 1 (PD-L1) expression (2%). The pleural drainage was subsequently removed and a suture applied.

Discussion Topic

Oncologist

In an 80-year-old patient, the side effects of polychemotherapy can be serious.

Pulmonologist

Could he benefit from radiation therapy?

Radiation oncologist

The lesion we confirmed histologically is the one located in the apical anterior area of the right upper lung lobe. However, two other lung lesions are highly suspicious. One is in the right upper lobe as well, and the other is in the left upper lung lobe.

Oncologist

Both have a low standardized uptake value (SUV); however, they don't look like inflammatory lesions at all. They were present on previous CT scans and now appear more compact.

Radiation oncologist

We can perform a CT simulation, without contrast medium, to study the feasibility of radiation therapy.

Oncologist

If radiation therapy is not feasible, we can propose palliative single-agent treatment.

The patient underwent CT simulation for planning of radiation therapy. The volume to be irradiated was considerable, and such treatment would have had an excessive risk of toxicity. Thus the doctors excluded radiation therapy and proposed single-agent treatment with gemcitabine.

Recommended Therapy and Further Indications at Discharge

After 9 days of hospitalization, the patient was discharged with the diagnosis of lung LPA. Single-agent treatment with gemcitabine was scheduled (1000 mg/m^2 on days 1 and 8, every 3 weeks, for four cycles).

Follow-Up and Outcomes

The patient underwent restaging with PET/CT after 3 and 6 months. Progression of disease was observed; in particular, all of the lung lesions had increased in size and in SUV value, and the lesion located anteriorly in the apical area of the right upper lobe also had colliquative–necrotic features (Fig. 20.6). Immunotherapy with nivolumab was subsequently proposed.

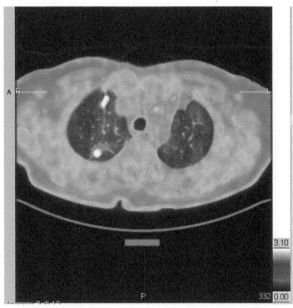

Fig. 20.6 Positron emission tomography/computed tomography (PET/CT) restaging after 6 months. An increase in the size and metabolic activity of the lesions in the right upper lung lobe are evident.

Focus On

Transthoracic Needle Aspiration and Biopsy

Transthoracic needle aspiration (TTNA) and biopsy (TTNB) are diagnostic techniques used to achieve a definitive diagnosis of pleural or lung lesions. Lesion localization can be defined under the guidance of computed tomography (CT) or ultrasonography just before the procedure. No premedication is routinely administered to the patient. Laboratory blood tests, including platelet count, prothrombin time, and international normalized ratio (INR), are required before the procedure.

Usually, TTNA uses 18-, 20-, or 22-gauge needles. TTNB involves percutaneous insertion of a hollow large-bore needle (usually 18-gauge), with a specially adapted cutting mechanism (Tru-cut needle), to extract a piece of tissue (core biopsy). Biopsy or aspiration materials are fixed in alcohol and sent for pathological examination. Immediate cytological evaluation increases the diagnostic yield. However, in many centers, it is difficult to ensure the presence of a pathologist during the examination.

Chest CT or radiography is indicated immediately after the procedure. Further imaging should be performed 4 to 6 hours later, particularly in patients at high risk for pneumothorax.

With both TTNA and TBNA, morbidity is limited and mortality is rare. Compared with TTNA, lung TTNB seems to achieve higher diagnostic accuracy with only a slightly higher complication risk.

Focus On

Complications of Transthoracic Needle Aspiration and Transthoracic Needle Biopsy

Pneumothorax is one of the most common complications of transthoracic needle aspiration (TTNA) or biopsy (TTNB) and usually occurs during or immediately after the procedure. Therefore, chest CT or radiography is performed soon after TTNA or TTNB. Additional erect chest radiography is required if pain, dyspnea, or hypoxemia develop, and in any case 4 to 6 hours after the procedure because delayed pneumothorax may also occur, sometimes necessitating chest tube insertion.

Available studies on adults who underwent TTNA or TTNB for lung nodules suggest an approximately 15% risk of pneumothorax. Less than half the cases of pneumothorax requires pleural drainage (overall, it is needed in 5%–10% of procedures). Older age (> 60 years), smoking, and chronic obstructive pulmonary disease (COPD) increase the risk for pneumothorax as a complication of CT-guided lung biopsy.

Further minor complications of the procedures include transient hemoptysis and pulmonary hemorrhage, which appears as ground-glass opacity around the target lesion. The incidence rate of hemorrhage is estimated to be around 1%; usually, no treatment is required.

Finally, air embolism and needle tract seeding are rare complications of TTNA and TTNB.

Focus On

Pleural Drainage and Techniques for Chest Tube Insertion

The insertion of a chest tube can be performed at the bedside for most patients.

Small- and medium-bore chest tubes are typically placed by using the Seldinger technique (catheter over guide wire) or through an atraumatic stylet that introduces the drain into the pleural space without the use of a guidewire. These are the most widespread methods because of ease of insertion and increased patient comfort. Large-bore (> 24-French [Fr]) chest tubes can be inserted via blunt dissection or by using the trocar technique, which is obsolete now.

The Seldinger technique uses a guidewire that is inserted into the pleural space through an introducer needle; the wire should pass without resistance. Then the needle is removed, and dilators can be passed over the wire by using a slight twisting action (tissue dilation is not always required). Subsequently, the chest tube is threaded over the guidewire to easily reach the pleural space. Finally, the wire guide is removed, and the tube is sutured to the skin. This technique may be used for both small and large chest tubes. Its main advantages are the smaller incision and minimal tissue dissection, resulting in less pain and reduced scar after removal of the drain. However, this technique makes it more difficult to direct the tube to the desired location of the pleural space.

New small-bore catheters are placed over their own rigid introducers. Usually, the introducer consists of a stylet with a spring-loaded covered tip that retracts during the initial compression on the outer surface of the thoracic wall, thus revealing the cutting edge of the needle (Verres-type needle). As soon as the introducer reaches the pleural space, the protective stylet returns once again to the extended position, thus protecting any underlying structures from damage. The entrance into the cavity may be accompanied by a clicking noise as a result of activation of the spring. Many kits also have an indicator that changes color when resistance is lost. Aspiration of air or fluid by the syringe confirms correct placement of the chest drain. While the chest tube is advanced into the pleural space, the stylet is removed. Finally, the chest tube is secured and connected to a one-way valve and a collection bag or drainage system.

In the trocar technique, a sharp-tipped rod (the trocar) is passed through the chest tube and then used to pierce the pleural space. An incision in the skin and subcutaneous tissue aids in inserting the trocar/tube combination into the pleural space. The chest tube is left in the pleural space and the trocar withdrawn. Although technically simple, this technique should be avoided because it has a high risk of complications, including misplaced drains and organ perforation.

Blunt dissection is the oldest technique for chest tube insertion. It is still performed for large-bore chest tubes (> 24-Fr). After administration of a local anesthetic, an incision is made in the skin and subcutaneous tissue, parallel to the rib. With the help of a clamp, the subcutaneous tissue and the intercostal muscles are dissected above the rib. Then the distal end of the chest tube is introduced into the pleural space.

The main advantages of such technique are the ability to perform digital exploration of the pleural space to assess for pleural adherences and to direct the tube into the most appropriate position within the thoracic cavity. Nevertheless, this method requires a larger incision compared with others; consequently, it is more painful and leaves a bigger scar after the tube is removed.

LEARNING POINTS

- Complications of CT-guided lung biopsy include early and delayed pneumothorax.
- In CT-guided lung biopsy, complications occur more often with core biopsy than with TTNA.
- Risk factors for TTNA and TTNB complications include smaller nodule diameter, larger needle diameter, and increased traversed lung parenchyma.
- Pleural drainage can be required in worsening pneumothorax after CT-guided lung biopsy.
- In most patients, chest tube placement can be performed at the bedside.
- Blunt dissection and trocar technique should be used only in selected cases and for large-bore chest tube placement because of their high risk of complications.

Further Reading

1. Choi CM, Um SW, Yoo CG, et al. Incidence and risk factors of delayed pneumothorax after transthoracic needle biopsy of the lung. *Chest.* 2004;126(5):1516–1521.
2. Zafar N, Dilip K, Sorino C. Transthoracic needle biopsy. In: Sorino C, editor. *Diagnostic Evaluation of the Respiratory System.* New Delhi: Jaypee Brothers Medical Publishers; 2017.
3. Heerink WJ, de Bock GH, de Jonge GJ, et al. Complication rates of CT-guided transthoracic lung biopsy: meta-analysis. *Eur Radiol.* 2017;27:138–148.
4. Porcel JM. Chest tube drainage of the pleural space: a concise review for pulmonologists. *Tuberc Respir Dis (Seoul).* 2018;81(2):106–115.
5. Wiener RS, Schwartz LM, Woloshin S, Welch HG. Population-based risk for complications after transthoracic needle lung biopsy of a pulmonary nodule: an analysis of discharge records. *Ann Intern Med.* 2011;155:137–144.

CHAPTER 21

Primary Spontaneous Right Pneumothorax in a Patient With Pulmonary Bullae

Claudio Sorino ■ Filippo Lococo ■ Stefano Negri ■ Stefano Elia
■ Giampietro Marchetti

History of Present Illness

A 35-year-old Caucasian man presented to the emergency room with sudden worsening of breathlessness, right chest pain, and dry cough.

Past Medical History

He worked as a construction engineer and was a current smoker (20 cigarettes/day). He had no previous exposure to noxious substances and no history of alcohol abuse or drug use. No allergies were known.

He had previous surgery for repair of testicular torsion and traumatic fracture of the humerus resulting from a traffic accident. There was no history of lung disease. In the past month, he had traveled by plane twice for work and had a little cough without fever or sputum.

Physical Examination and Early Clinical Findings

In the emergency room, the patient was found to be alert, cooperative, afebrile (body temperature 36.5° C [97.7° F]). Oxygen saturation (SpO$_2$), measured with pulse oximetry, was 90% while the patient was breathing ambient air. Heart rate was 98 beats/min, respiratory rate was 22 breaths/min, and blood pressure was 140/85 mm Hg. Electrocardiography (ECG) showed sinus tachycardia.

At the physical examination of the lungs, expansion of the right hemithorax was found to be reduced. On this side, reduction of breath sounds and hyperresonance to percussion at the upper field were evident. The remainder of the examination was normal.

The arterial blood gas (ABG) analysis on room air revealed acute respiratory failure (pH 7.44; partial pressure of carbon dioxide [PaCO$_2$] 35 mm Hg; partial pressure of oxygen [PaO$_2$] 55 mm Hg; bicarbonate [HCO$_3^-$] 24 mmol/L); therefore oxygen therapy was started.

Blood tests showed mild leukocytosis (white blood cell [WBC] count was 9,940/mm^3 with normal differential count); C-reactive protein (CRP) was 19.7 mg/L (normal values < 5 mg/L); and hemoglobin (Hb) was 16.1 g/dL. Cardiac enzymes (troponin and creatine kinase MB) were not altered.

Point-of-care ultrasonography of the chest showed absence of pleural sliding, but no clear lung point.

Chest radiography revealed right pneumothorax extending from the apex to the base, without a significant mediastinal shift (Fig. 21.1).

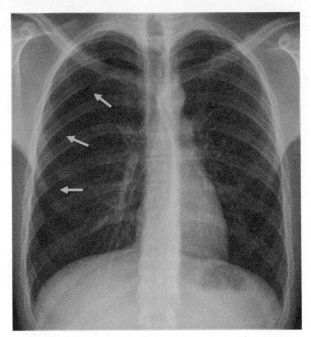

Fig. 21.1 Posteroanterior chest radiograph showing right pneumothorax with partial lung collapse. The visceral pleural edge is seen as a very thin, sharp white line *(yellow arrows)*. The peripheral space is radiolucent and without lung markings.

Discussion Topic

Radiologist

The patient has large right pneumothorax. It extends from the apex to the base of the hemithorax. The mediastinum is not displaced.

ER doctor

Is the lung completely collapsed?

Radiologist

No, it isn't. However, the distance from the chest wall is greater than 3 cm. It was not necessary to get a radiograph in expiration.

Pulmonologist

This is already an indication for needle aspiration or placement of a thoracic drain.

Discussion Topic—cont'd

ER doctor

Can we perform immediately a chest computed tomography (CT) to better visualize the lung parenchyma?

Pulmonologist

The patient has respiratory failure, and we need to promptly remove air from the pleural space to achieve lung reexpansion. I suggest performing CT after the procedure.

ER doctor

I agree, clinical conditions could rapidly deteriorate.

Clinical Course

The pulmonologist prepared for placing a chest tube. Platelet count and the international normalized ratio (INR) were acceptable. The patient was informed about the importance of the procedure and the potential risks and was able to provide signed informed consent. A single dose of prophylactic antibiotic (cefazolin 1 g intravenous) was administered. Trichotomy of the thoracic surface and skin disinfection were performed. After filling a syringe with lidocaine, the pulmonologist inserted the needle into the second right intercostal space, along the hemiclavicular line. The local anesthetic was injected into the subcutaneous tissue, then more deeply until air bubbles coming from the pleural cavity were evident inside the syringe. Subsequently, a small incision was made with a scalpel, and an 18-French (Fr) pleural drain was placed (Fig. 21.2). The tube was connected to a collection chamber, and air immediately came out from the pleural space. The patient got relief from breathlessness. He was admitted to the pulmonology department for continuation of treatment and monitoring of the pleural drainage.

Discussion Topic

ER doctor

Wasn't needle aspiration enough? Why did you place a chest tube?

Pulmonologist

The pneumothorax is probably caused by rupture of subpleural blebs or bullae. Chest drainage allows for determining if the air leakage persists and for preventing hypertension pneumothorax. A small-bore tube is usually adequate for this.

Continued

Discussion Topic—cont'd

ER doctor

In the case of pneumothorax, do you always insert the tube anteriorly?

Pulmonologist

The second or third intercostal space at the midclavicular line is only one of the possible insertion site. In patients with very thick chest walls, you can insert the chest tube in the so-called safety triangle, usually in the fifth intercostal space, along the midaxillary line.

ER doctor

Will the patient continue to receive antibiotics after tube placement to prevent pleural or lung infections?

Pulmonologist

No, he won't. Actually, antibiotics are not strictly needed when a chest tube is placed for spontaneous pneumothorax.

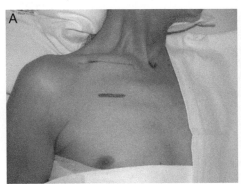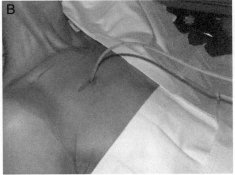

Fig. 21.2 (A) Identification of the insertion point of the thoracic tube in the second right intercostal space along the hemiclavicular line. (B) pleural drainage in place (stitches not yet applied).

During the subsequent days, the patient did not have shortness of breath or cough. He asked for an analgesic (paracetamol) only a few times because of pain at the site of chest tube insertion. SpO_2 increased to 99% with low oxygen support (fraction of inspired oxygen [FiO_2]: 28%). However, there was continuous air leakage through the thoracic drainage. Chest computed tomography (CT) showed only partial resolution of the right pneumothorax and the presence of peripheral lung bullae (Fig. 21.3). Therefore the thoracic surgeon proposed bullectomy through uniportal video-assisted thoracic surgery (U-VATS) (Fig. 21.4).

Discussion Topic

Pulmonologist

The patient continues to have air leakage through the chest tube. Do you think we should wait and see what happens in the next few days, or should we proceed differently?

Thoracic surgeon

Chest CT showed at least one subpleural bubble. It is advisable to inspect the lung surface and probably carry out bullectomy to prevent recurrences.

Pulmonologist

Do you recommend surgical thoracoscopy?

Thoracic surgeon

Yes, I have good experience with the uniportal technique. I should be able to perform the procedure with a single access port.

Pulmonologist

Can you give me some suggestions on antibiotic prophylaxis in case of thoracic surgery?

Thoracic surgeon

When video-assisted thoracoscopic surgery (VATS) or thoracotomy is required, you can give cephalosporin, such as intravenous cefazolin 1 to 2 g in a single dose, or every 8 hours up to three doses. Studies have shown that in noncardiac thoracic surgery, there is no clinically significant benefit in using antibiotics longer than 24 hours.

Cefepime is preferable in patients who are at risk for high anaerobic burden, for example, as a result of perforation, because it has better anaerobic coverage.

A common scheme is cefepime 1 g prior to incision, followed by three doses, each given every 12 hours.

Pulmonologist

Thanks. And what do you do if patients have a history of methicillin-resistant *Staphylococcus aureus* (MRSA) infection or a penicillin allergy?

Thoracic surgeon

If the patient is at risk for MRSA infection, you can add a glycopeptide antibiotic, such as intravenous vancomycin 500 mg every 6 hours for a total of three doses. In patients with penicillin allergy, you can use a fluoroquinolone instead of a cephalosporin, for example levofloxacin 500 mg every 12 hours for a total of three doses.

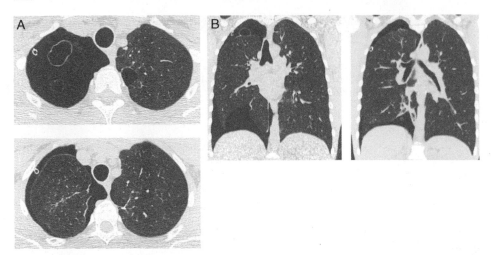

Fig. 21.3 Chest computed tomography (CT) scan showing residual right pneumothorax despite pleural drainage and peripheral lung bullae. (A) Axial plane. (B) Coronal plane.

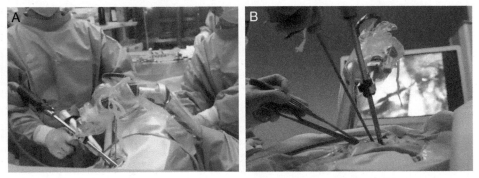

Fig. 21.4 Uniportal video-assisted thoracic surgery (VATS). (A) Panoramic view. (B) Instruments.

On hospital day 7, the patient underwent thoracic surgery. General anesthesia was provided through a double-lumen tube to maintain single-lung ventilation. A plastic wound protector was used for the operation port incision. U-VATS showed a large dystrophic area with several bullae in the apex of the right lung (Fig. 21.5). The water submersion test revealed a large air leak at this level. The bullae were resected, and selective chemical pleurodesis with talc in the pulmonary apex and mechanical pleurodesis in the entire chest cavity was performed to reduce recurrences. A 24-Fr pleural drainage was placed in the posterior–basal thoracic area. Intravenous cefazolin 1 g was administrated before the incision and then every 8 hours for a total of three doses. The postoperative course was uncomplicated.

Recommended Therapy and Further Indications at Discharge

The patient was discharged 4 days after VATS. No home therapy was prescribed, except for paracetamol as needed. Close outpatient follow-up after hospital discharge was recommended.

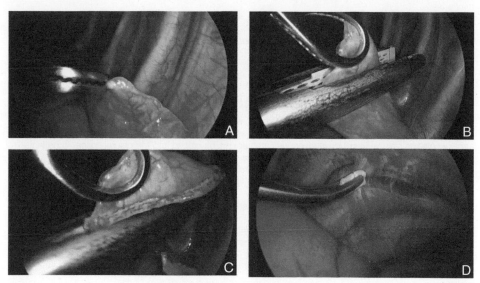

Fig. 21.5 Direct visualization of the right lung apex during video-assisted thoracic surgery (VATS). (A) Identification of some bubbles. (B and C) Mechanical staple bullectomy. (D) Pleural abrasion for mechanical pleurodesis.

Follow-Up and Outcomes

The patient was re-evaluated on an outpatient basis 10 and 20 days after VATS. The stitches were removed, and chest radiography showed maintenance of good lung expansion. There was no recurrence of pneumothorax during the subsequent 8 months of follow-up.

Focus On

Spontaneous Pneumothorax

Pneumothorax is described as spontaneous when it is not caused by trauma or any obvious precipitating factor.

Primary spontaneous pneumothorax (PSP) occurs in people without clinically apparent lung disease. It usually occurs at rest, in individuals younger than 20 years of age, and rarely in those older than 40 years of age. The main risk factors for PSP are cigarette smoking, family history, Marfan syndrome, and homocystinuria. Cases of PSP are described in patients with severe malnutrition caused by anorexia nervosa.

Secondary spontaneous pneumothorax (SSP) is a complication of pre-existing lung disease. About 50% to 70% of SSP cases are attributed to chronic obstructive pulmonary disease (COPD). Patients with apical blebs and severe bronchial obstruction have the greatest risk for SSP. Other causes include cystic fibrosis, lung malignancy, pneumonia, tuberculous cavities, and thoracic endometriosis.

Most individuals with PSP have unrecognized lung disease, with pneumothorax resulting from rupture of a subpleural bleb.

The clinical presentation depends on the size of pneumothorax, rapidity of onset, tension within the pleural space, patient's age, and severity of the underlying lung disease.

Focus On

Management of Primary Spontaneous Pneumothorax

Early management of primary spontaneous pneumothorax (PSP) mainly depends on patient features and clinical presentation.

Supplemental oxygen and observation can be reserved for patients experiencing their first episode of PSP and who are clinically stable and have small pneumothorax ($\leq$ 3 cm between the lung and the chest wall, as seen on a chest radiograph).

Patients with large pneumothorax (> 3 cm) or with symptoms, such as chest pain or dyspnea, should undergo needle aspiration or small-bore chest tube placement to remove air from the pleural space. Alternatively, a 14-gauge intravenous catheter can be placed into the pleural space. In patients with thick chest walls, needles or catheters as long as 7 cm may be needed.

Preferred insertion sites are the second or the third intercostal space (ICS) at the midclavicular line (in patients without very thick chest walls) and the fifth ICS between the anterior axillary line and the midaxillary line.

The chest tube is usually connected to a water seal device rather than to a Heimlich valve. Suction should be avoided because of the risk of re-expansion pulmonary edema but can be considered if the pneumothorax fails to resolve.

Once the lung has expanded, if the air leakage has resolved, the chest tube can be removed.

Thoracoscopy is indicated in case of recurrent PSP or hemopneumothorax or when air leakage persists after chest tube insertion, even if the patient is clinically stable.

Focus On

Uniportal Versus Multiport Video-Assisted Thoracoscopic Surgery for Anatomical Lung Resections

In the past, open thoracotomy was the only way to access the thoracic cavity. Advances in thoracic surgery have led to the development of less invasive thoracoscopic procedures. Video-assisted thoracoscopic surgery (VATS) was introduced in the 1990s and has been subsequently used increasingly for pulmonary resections both in lung cancer and other nonneoplastic lung diseases.

About half the pulmonary resections are performed through VATS. The potential benefits of VATS include smaller incisions, reduced postoperative pain, lower rate of complications, and shorter hospital stays.

Many oncologic studies have shown similar results, including survival rates, for patients undergoing VATS lobectomy and conventional lobectomy through open thoracotomy.

Multiport VATS requires multiple small incisions in the chest wall, allowing introduction of a video camera and surgical instruments into the thoracic cavity. In the past 20 years, three-port VATS has evolved to two-port VATS and subsequently to uniportal VATS. The last is performed increasingly more because of the advantages associated with the breach of only a single intercostal space while guaranteeing a view similar to that of open surgery for the surgeon.

LEARNING POINTS

- The rupture of subpleural blebs or bullae is a common cause of spontaneous pneumothorax.
- Large pneumothorax (>3 cm) or with symptoms should undergo needle aspiration or chest tube placement.
- Thoracoscopy is indicated in case of recurrent PSP, hemopneumothorax, or when air leak persists after chest tube insertion.

Further Reading

1. MacDuff A, Arnold A, Harvey J BTS Pleural Disease Guideline Group. Management of spontaneous pneumothorax: British Thoracic Society Pleural Disease Guideline 2010. *Thorax*. 2010;65(Suppl 2):ii18–31.
2. Sahn SA, Heffner JE. Spontaneous pneumothorax. *N Engl J Med*. 2000;342(12):868–874.
3. Noppen M, De Keukeleire T. Pneumothorax. *Respiration*. 2008;76(2):121–127.
4. Tschopp JM, Rami-Porta R, Noppen M, Astoul P. Management of spontaneous pneumothorax: state of the art. *Eur Respir J*. 2006;28(3):637–650.
5. Light RW. Pleural controversy: optimal chest tube size for drainage. *Respirology*. 2011;16(2):244–248.
6. Shaikhrezai K, Thompson AI, Parkin C, et al. Video-assisted thoracoscopic surgery management of spontaneous pneumothorax-long-term results. *Eur J Cardiothorac Surg*. 2011;40(1):120–123.
7. Erşen E, Kılıç B, Kara HV, et al. Uniportal versus multiport video-assisted thoracoscopic surgery for anatomical lung resections: a glance at a dilemma. *Wideochir Inne Tech Maloinwazyjne*. 2018;13(2):215–220.
8. Nachira D, Ismail M, Meacci E. Uniportal vs. triportal video-assisted thoracic surgery in the treatment of primary pneumothorax—a propensity matched bicentric study. *J Thorac Dis*. 2018;10(Suppl 31):S3712–S3719.
9. Chang SH, Krupnick AS. Perioperative antibiotics in thoracic surgery. *Thorac Surg Clin*. 2012;22(1):35–45.

Page numbers followed by "*b*," "*f*," and "*t*" indicate boxes, figures, and tables, respectively.